ROGERS JAMES SEYMOUR is a former CPR instructor-trainer for the American Heart Association. He is also a consultant for setting up CPR programs in schools and has taught CPR techniques to hundreds of interested learners.

ROGERS JAMES SEYMOUR

THE HEART ATTACK SURVIVAL MANUAL

A Guide to Using CPR
(Cardiopulmonary Resuscitation)
in a Crisis

8105̄70

A SPECTRUM BOOK

PRENTICE-HALL, INC., Englewood Cliffs, New Jersey 07632

BORDENTOWN BRANCH
BURLINGTON COUNTY LIBRARY
BORDENTOWN, NJ 08505

Library of Congress Cataloging in Publication Data

Seymour, Rogers James.
  The heart attack survival manual.

  (A Spectrum Book)
  Bibliography: p.
  1. Heart—Infarction. 2. Resuscitation. I. Title.
[DNLM: 1. Heart arrest—Therapy. 2. Resuscitation.
WG205 S521h]
RC685.I6S46   616.1'230252   80-20317
ISBN 0-13-385740-9
ISBN 0-13-385732-8 (pbk.)

For Raymond Frank Seymour

© 1981 by Prentice-Hall, Inc., Englewood Cliffs, New Jersey 07632

A SPECTRUM BOOK

All rights reserved. No part of this book may be reproduced in any form or by any means without permission in writing from the publisher.

10   9   8   7   6   5   4   3   2   1

Printed in the United States of America

Editorial/production supervision and interior design by Frank Moorman
Cover design by Honi Werner
Manufacturing buyer: Barbara A. Frick

PRENTICE-HALL INTERNATIONAL, INC., *London*
PRENTICE-HALL OF AUSTRALIA PTY. LIMITED, *Sydney*
PRENTICE-HALL OF CANADA, LTD., *Toronto*
PRENTICE-HALL OF INDIA PRIVATE LIMITED, *New Delhi*
PRENTICE-HALL OF JAPAN, INC., *Tokyo*
PRENTICE-HALL OF SOUTHEAST ASIA PTE. LTD., *Singapore*
WHITEHALL BOOKS LIMITED, *Wellington, New Zealand*

BORDENTOWN BRANCH
BURLINGTON COUNTY LIBRARY
BORDENTOWN, NJ 08505

Contents

Foreword by Denton A. Cooley, M.D., v

1. Epidemic, 1

2. CPR: taking a life in your hands, 5

3. CPR works, 9

4. Learning CPR, 13

5. What happens when a heart stops, 17

6. Detecting a heart attack, 23

7. Getting help, 31

8. Learning the ABCs, 37

9. Questions and answers about CPR, 59

10. Two-person rescues, 71

11. CPR for infants and small children, 79

12. A quick review, 89

13. Good Samaritan laws, 91

14. How to save your own life, 93

15. Telling others about CPR, 103

16. Attending a CPR class, 107

Bibliography, 111

Foreword

Several months ago I deboarded an afternoon plane at the Houston Intercontinental Airport and proceeded with the crowd of passengers down the long ramp to the main terminal. Lying facedown on the floor was an obese, elderly woman completely motionless with hand luggage cast aside—she was not breathing. Other passengers glanced briefly at her and then continued on their way, expressing curiosity but no apparent concern. I dropped my parcels and went to my knees beside her—her lips were purple, and her tongue was protruding between her teeth, saliva at the corners of her mouth. I quickly turned her onto her back, i.e., from the prone to the supine position. Not having a stethoscope, I placed my ear against her chest and could detect no heart sounds. How long had she been dead?

I compressed her chest wall three or four times and then established ventilation of her lungs. To do this I elevated her jaw (mandible) with the left hand and opened her lips with the other. Taking in a deep breath and with a wide open mouth pressed to hers, I blew into her salivating mouth. After three or four of these breaths for pulmonary ventilation, I again compressed her breast bone repeatedly until color returned to her lips and face. Within a few minutes she opened her eyes, looked around in wonderment at the small group of people around, and within fifteen minutes, was apparently normal. Her son, who was to meet her at the airport, arrived on the scene explaining that he had gone to the wrong gate and was feeling guilty for not being available to carry his 74-year-old mother's bags. A wheelchair was obtained, and he took her to a local hospital where she was scheduled for orthopedic surgery later in the week. I have never heard from her since, but imagine my spiritual exhilaration at having saved a life!

The experience made a lasting impression on me—not because of the miracle of cardiopulmonary resuscitation (CPR) that becomes almost routine to a cardiac surgeon—but because of the response or lack of response by others who had discovered the woman on the floor before I arrived. Why had they just walked by and not attempted to render aid? Several possibilities seem reasonable, such as reluctance to get involved, concern over personal liability and legal consequence, lack of compassion in a contemporary, impersonal society, and the inconvenience caused by involvement in a situation which could require valuable time in a hurried situation. But the factor which may be most important was *fear*—a fear growing out of ignorance. Perhaps some assumed that the woman was dead and could not bring themselves to touch a human corpse. Most people have little understanding of the definition or meaning of life and death. If the heart stops, is that death? If breathing stops . . . ? Is it proper from an ethical, religious, or legal standpoint to resurrect the dead? Disregarding the obvious significance of that type of ignorance and superstition, did the fear grow out of the average person's lack of knowledge about cardiopulmonary resuscitation? Had someone else in that airport obtained some knowledge of this method of revitalization, he could have accomplished the same feat. How often would a cardiac surgeon be available under such circumstances? The odds against that happening are astronomical. Yet lives can be saved under similar circumstances by informed or trained laymen. If the technique is applied too late or fails for other reasons, the person applying the treatment can have the consolation of saying, "I tried!"

Heart disease today is the major cause of death in the United States. Increasing emphasis is being placed upon prevention and treatment, and fortunately, recent statistics reveal that the death rate from heart disease has already declined slightly. Yet all of these measures, including proper exercise, diet, appropriate recreation, and work habits, will never eliminate sudden death. Many patients die from cardiac dysfunctions or conduction disturbances which are readily reversible by cardiopulmonary resuscitation. Even in those instances where some underlying more serious or permanent damage results, the maintenance of circulation and oxygenation of blood by CPR, while the victim is being transferred to a hospital or specialized coronary care unit, may prolong life for many years. Moreover, with the present day use of sophisticated diagnostic equipment, newer pharmacologic agents and drugs, temporary cardiac assist devices, and surgical repair by coronary artery bypass, cardiac valve replacement, implantation of electronic pacemakers, and so on, many patients are restored to a long and healthy life and lifestyle after major cardiac events. Thus one should recognize and appreciate the need for widespread dissemination of the knowledge imparted by Jim Seymour, author of *The Heart Attack Survival Manual,* who has extensive experience as an instructor in CPR. Perhaps you, the reader, can save a life, maybe of someone very close and dear to you.

Denton A. Cooley, MD.
Surgeon-in-Chief
Texas Heart Institute
Houston, Texas

1 Epidemic!

You're probably going to die of heart disease.

How can I say that? Because today, more than half of all deaths in the United States result from heart disease.

Not just in-hospital deaths. Not just the deaths of the elderly. Not just those deaths attributed to some form of "disease."

All deaths. Including those from car wrecks, shooting accidents, airplane crashes, knifings, poisoning, and every other category. *A majority of all deaths—more than a million a year— are caused by heart disease.*

So the odds are clear: You're probably going to die from heart disease.

Unless you—and we, as a society—do something about that grim statistic.

In 1975, the last year for which data are available, 53 percent

1

of all deaths in the United States resulted from what physicians call *cardiovascular disease.* About two-thirds of those deaths were from heart attacks, and more than half of those people were DOA at a hospital.

Think heart disease is less of a threat than cancer? *Three times as many people die from heart disease as from cancer.*

Think heart disease is restricted to the elderly? *One-fourth of all deaths from heart disease occur in persons under 65.*

Think you can beat those odds?

You can.

Because, while the United States (and many other developed nations) have been swept up in what the World Health Organization defines as a genuine "epidemic" of heart disease, we have also learned much more about what causes heart attacks and strokes—and how to avoid them.

And we have also learned how to save many, perhaps most, of those victims.

It's noontime; you're leaving your office building for lunch. As you step out of the elevator on the ground floor, one of your fellow passengers suddenly clutches his chest, utters a low groan, slumps to the floor. He is ashen, almost blue. People pull back in horror; some scream. Someone yells "Get an ambulance! This man . . . he . . . I think . . . it looks like a heart attack!"

Would you know what to do to save his life?

Or you're at home in the evening, curled up in front of the television. Your wife, who has been complaining of "gas" pains since dinner, frowns, grimaces, then cries out, "My chest! Ohhh, it hurts. I feel dizzy. I feel. . . ." She crumples, collapses on the floor. She is not breathing, and you can't find a pulse.

Would you know what to do to save her life?

Or you're on the golf course. Your lifelong friend, the one with the big handicap because he doesn't get to play much anymore since his big promotion, has been playing well. You've both won a few bucks. As he gets out of the electric cart you share, he swallows hard, complains of tightness in his chest, "a pulled muscle, I guess." He adds that he's been having "this damn pain on the inside of my arm all morning." Probably another pulled muscle.

He walks over to the ball, lines up the long two-iron shot, swings. He hits the ball well: As you follow it, you see it hit the green, run up within a few inches from the cup. "Not bad," you call out as you look back toward him, expecting to see that silly grin you know so well.

Except that he isn't grinning. He's lying on the ground, his club bent and broken, his eyes wide open, his skin almost white. One hand is clutching at his chest, right over the little alligator on his shirt.

He is not making a sound. He has stopped breathing. He has begun to die.

Would you know what to do to save his life?

Not so long ago—as recently as the early Sixties—there wouldn't have been much you could do to save any of those lives. Call an ambulance? Sure. But it takes at least several minutes for an ambulance to arrive—often much longer, especially in congested downtown areas, outlying suburbs, and in rural areas—and the fate of a heart attack victim is usually sealed in the first five minutes or so after an attack.

But there has been a dramatic change for the better.

Thanks to a technique known as *cardiopulmonary resuscitation*, usually called CPR, the lives of these victims and many, many more—perhaps a half million a year—can be saved by alert, trained bystanders. Like you.

Not a physician. Or a nurse.

You.

Because CPR, though an immensely powerful technique—just what a physician does for a heart attack victim away from elaborate medical facilities—is simple and easy to learn, perfectly suitable for lay persons' use.

You can learn how to do CPR.

You can learn how to save a life. Perhaps the life of someone you've never met, a stranger you may never see again. Or perhaps the life of your wife, or son, or neighbor, or business partner.

You can do it. You can learn CPR.

You'll be in good company.

In June 1977, the Gallup Organization polled Americans on their knowledge of and feelings about CPR. About two-thirds of all Americans had heard of CPR; more than half wanted to learn

CPR for themselves. And more than twelve million had already completed CPR courses.*

Many businesses and government agencies provide free CPR instruction for their employees. Students in junior and senior high schools in at least thirty-five states learn CPR as part of their regular schoolwork. Across the United States local chapters of the American Heart Association and Red Cross, YM and YWCAs, fire departments, rescue squads, Junior Leagues, and community groups of every sort offer CPR training.

Because it's important that *as many of us as possible learn this lifesaving skill.* You cannot perform CPR on yourself, only on another. So your best chance for help if you suffer a heart attack is that someone else nearby will know what to do, how to save your life with CPR. The larger the percentage of the population familiar with CPR, the more lives saved.

In the greater Seattle area, community groups set a goal of one person in five trained in CPR. A coordinated, communitywide effort met that goal in less than three years. Today the percentage of Seattle-area residents trained in CPR is even higher.

Are there some people who probably can't learn CPR?

If you've recently had a heart attack or open-heart surgery, you should probably defer learning and practicing CPR till your doctor gives you the go-ahead. If you have emphysema or other breathing difficulties, you might find CPR too tiring. If you're very tiny, very weak, or both, you may not be able to learn to do CPR. If you have any questions about whether CPR is something you should attempt, ask your doctor. You'll probably be told to go ahead—and be congratulated that you're learning CPR.

The evidence indicates that perhaps 95 percent of the population *can* learn CPR. In the author's experience—in training several hundred people to perform CPR, ranging in age from 14 to 87, including people with broken legs, one lung, histories of heart attacks, and even one woman confined to a wheelchair—almost anyone who *wants* to learn CPR *can* learn.

You can learn CPR.

You can learn how to take a life in your hands.
And save it.

---

*Poll data, copyright 1977, Field Enterprises, Inc.

2 CPR: taking a life in your hands

Though it is a simple skill, performed without any instruments or other tools beyond one's own hands and mouth, CPR seems sophisticated, compared to earlier means of saving victims of heart attacks and other forms of sudden death.

Death looks like sleep, so through the ages man has tried to deal with it as he would with an especially deep sleep. Slapping victims, dousing them with hot or cold water, whipping them with stinging nettles, making loud noises, even building fires atop victims' abdomens were all tried. Without success.

Early American colonists were told by their new Indian friends that tobacco smoke had certain magic powers, including the capacity to revive the dead. The colonists adopted the Indians' procedure of blowing tobacco smoke up victim's anuses to revive them; the Dutch, English, and others also adopted the technique. But only briefly, for it did not work.

On wharfs all over the world seamen rolled drowning and other sudden-death victims back and forth over barrels or threw them across trotting horses, in an effort to get the heart going, the lungs working. This actually worked in some cases—it is very roughly analogous to what we do in CPR—and is still used in some remote areas.

In the sixteenth century experiments using fireplace bellows to blow air into victims were reported, with occasional success.

In 1745 an English surgeon, William Tossach, told a meeting of colleagues of his success in reviving a suffocating coal miner by mouth-to-mouth breathing. He said it was a "vulgar" technique; but it had worked.

From the mid-1800s through the late 1930s, methods involving pulling on a victim's arms, pressing on his back, and other physical manipulation of the body became popular. Probably the best-known of these, the Schaeffer Prone-Pressure Method, involved a rescuer kneeling astride a prone, face-down victim. Pressure applied to the back pressed the abdomen against the diaphragm, causing an exhaling action; release of the pressure (later accompanied by lifting the arms, in the Holger-Nielsen Method) encouraged inhalation.

All of these later methods worked—sometimes.

The development of modern cardiopulmonary resuscitation is generally credited to researchers at Johns Hopkins University Medical School in Baltimore. During the late 1950s several researchers elsewhere had shown the superiority of mouth-to-mouth breathing over the older Holger-Nielsen Method; the Johns Hopkins team combined this with their new external cardiac compression technique to provide both *artificial respiration* and *artificial circulation*. For the first time, heart attack victims could get not only an air exchange, bringing vital oxygen, but also a simulated pumping action over their hearts, to deliver it, via the blood, to the oxygen-starved tissue in the brain and elsewhere.

Artificial Respiration + Artificial Circulation = CPR

The first success of the new technique drew worldwide attention. A Baltimore City Fire Department emergency rescue squad, trained in the new method by the Johns Hopkins team, answered a call only to find a man, just home from the hospital from an earlier heart attack, in cardiac arrest.

They performed mouth-to-mouth breathing and external chest compression while transporting him to Johns Hopkins. Twenty-three minutes after they began, a physician applied an electrical shock to his chest, and his heart began beating normally again. A month later the man left the hospital, the first heart attack victim saved by the new technique.

Because of the dangers and apparent complexity of the chest compression technique, it was at first assumed that only physicians, nurses, and perhaps emergency medical aides could be taught to perform it without greater danger to the victim. In September 1962, the American Heart Association issued a statement declaring that because of the hazards of chest compression, training of lay persons should be "limited to pilot programs only."

But field experience and those first, pioneering pilot programs soon showed that lay persons could be taught to perform CPR safely and competently. By 1974 the Heart Association was recommending that "CPR training be given to all eighth-grade pupils, and that it be repeated every year through high school."

Although we have so far referred to the use of CPR only in terms of saving victims of heart attacks, it should be emphasized that CPR also saves lives in cases of drowning, severe electrical shock, adverse drug reactions, smoke inhalation, stroke, and many other emergencies; in fact, the same technique is used any time a victim has stopped breathing and/or his heart has stopped.

In every case the procedure is just the same: the same steps, in the same order, will give victims of these life-threatening emergencies the same chance for life heart attack victims enjoy when a bystander performs CPR.

3 CPR works!

How many heart attack victims' lives could be saved if everyone knew CPR?

No one knows.

Over the past dozen years many studies have been reported in the professional medical journals, covering research into the effectiveness of CPR. Because of the many variables—studies covering in-hospital versus out-of-hospital attacks, different standards for classifying "cardiac events," enormous differences in lay CPR-training programs, varying bystander response time, and other critical determinants—no single study has given us an absolute answer to the question: How many lives can be saved with CPR?

But one careful study, published in the December 1977 issue of the journal *Circulation*, probably comes closest to giving a simple, authoritative answer to our question.

Dr. Donald Copley and others on staff at the Coronary Care Unit of the University of Alabama Medical Center in Birmingham did a detailed retrospective study of nineteen consecutive patients admitted following heart attacks.

Of the nineteen victims, seven had received quick, effective CPR from a bystander within five minutes after their attack. The other twelve got no help until an ambulance arrived and paramedics took over. (These patients received resuscitation assistance too, of course, from the paramedics, but not until more than five minutes after the attack.)

Of the seven victims who got quick CPR from a bystander, five lived and were judged unchanged from their preattack condition; one lived but had memory impairment; and one died. (Interestingly, the one fatality occurred in a victim who did not get CPR until almost five minutes after the attack. The others received help more quickly.)

What of the twelve who received no resuscitation assistance until arrival of emergency units? Six died, five lived but had central nervous system damage, and only one survivor was judged unchanged from preattack condition.

Of those who got quick CPR, six of seven survived. Of those who did not, half died, and five of the six survivors had central nervous system damage.

Figure 3-1

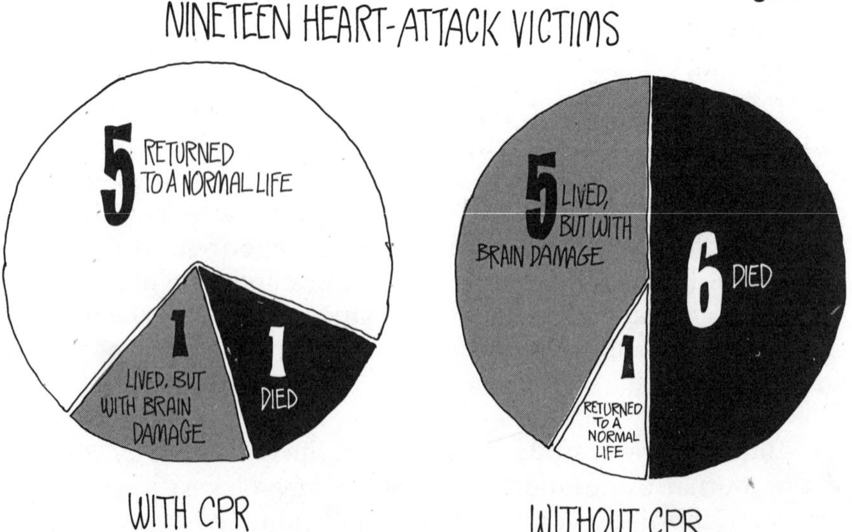

NINETEEN HEART-ATTACK VICTIMS

WITH CPR   WITHOUT CPR

Does that mean we can save five or six out of every seven heart attack victims with widespread CPR instruction? We do not yet know. But the Birmingham study, and others, clearly show that many, probably most, heart attack victims *can* be saved.

Other studies elsewhere offer further encouragement.

In Belfast, Northern Ireland, Dr. J. F. Pantridge coordinated a project which showed that 62 percent of those persons receiving CPR within the first four minutes after an attack survived. In Oslo, Norway, Drs. Ivar Lund and Andreas Skulberg reported a large-scale study which showed that even with many mistakes in their rescue techniques, lay persons were able to save the lives of more than a third of those who received bystander-initiated CPR; when that help was provided within the first minute after the attack, the percentage of successful "saves" increased to 61 percent.

Some reports have indicated the long-term survival rate of those resuscitated through CPR may be "only" about 20 percent. But these studies, focusing on those persons alive months or years after their rescue, ignore many others who survived the initial attack thanks to quick, effective CPR but later died from a second or later heart attack or even from other causes.

It is clear that the percentage of successful "saves" with CPR is closely related to the percentage of persons in an area who are knowledgeable in CPR. With increasing numbers of Seattle-area residents trained in CPR, the percentage of "saves" among out-of-hospital heart attacks there increased more than two and a half times, from less than one in ten to about one in four.

And all around us we have evidence of the success of CPR.

Judge John Sirica, famed for his handling of many of the defendants in the Watergate scandals, suffered a devastating heart attack while addressing a bar association luncheon. Quick work by a young Justice Department aide saved his life.

Texas Rangers pitcher "Doc" Medich, a surgical resident who learned CPR in medical school, has twice saved heart attack victims who collapsed at baseball games.

At Marineland, in California, three high school students saved the life of a young woman held under water almost four minutes by a jealous killer whale.

In Mankato, Minnesota, Sara Haskell and Steve Meyer were getting married. A guest at their wedding, Sara's great-great aunt, collapsed in the church. Sara and her maid of honor, Deb Raines, both knew CPR: they stopped the ceremony, went to work . . . and saved Aunt Amy's life. (P.S.: The ceremony resumed, and Sara is now Mrs. Steve Meyer.)

Sammy Piner, an Atlantic Beach, North Carolina, policeman, pulled Maria Brown off the beach after she suffered a direct hit from a lightning bolt. She was badly burned, was not breathing, had no pulse. He immediately began CPR, soon aided by another bystander. By the time the ambulance arrived a few minutes later, her heart had resumed beating and she was breathing on her own. Later, lightning-strike expert Dr. Helen Taussig told reporters, "The overwhelming probability is that an accident of that kind is fatal—*unless* someone on the spot administers CPR. . . ."

In Pennington, New Jersey, Mrs. Marianne Cox took a CPR course, sure she'd never really need to use it. Just ten days later she pulled her two-year-old son Danny from a swimming pool, "cold and clammy," apparently drowned. She used CPR to save his life.

In Seattle, David Hansen has "died" twice. The first time, a co-worker, Niels Hansen, saved his life; the second time it was a newsstand operator, Earl Hatch. Seattle neighbor Harold Maxum's wife has saved his life *three* times with CPR.

And in Lake Worth, Florida, a funeral attendant trained in CPR actually "brought back" Buck Lawrence, a sixty-eight-year-old retired banker . . . after a doctor had declared Lawrence legally dead!

The stories could go on and on. Thousands of lives have been saved by lay persons who knew what to do, and *did* it, when someone around them collapsed with a heart attack or was pulled lifeless from a swimming pool or was found lying across a high-voltage line.

These rescuers aren't supermen, and they're not medical professionals. They're ordinary people, like you, like your neighbors.

And the moral of these stories is simple: You can do it, too. You can learn how to save a life.

4 Learning CPR

This book can tell you all the whys and hows of CPR. When you finish it, you'll probably know more about CPR than many persons who teach CPR day-in, day-out.

But what this book cannot do—what no book can do—is give you the experience of having performed, having practiced, CPR yourself. And since CPR is what psychologists call a "psychomotor skill," learned only by hands-on practice, that experience is essential.

Actual practice, on a specially designed CPR-training manni-kin, is an absolute must for becoming proficient at CPR.

Don't decide that a quick once-over of this book—or even careful study—equips you to use this lifesaving skill. A careful reading can prepare you to breeze through a CPR course in your community in much less time than other students. And you'll probably be a much more competent rescuer than those without benefit of the book. But no one should attempt to perform CPR without first completing a practice session with a CPR-training mannikin.

Please don't think you can get that necessary practice by experimenting upon a friend.

Go up to your spouse and tell him, "Come here George, and lie down on the floor a minute; I want to show you something I've been reading about"—and George may never get up again.

We never practice CPR on someone who does not need it. To do so can cause grievous injury, perhaps even death.

Remember: No human practice!

How, then, do you go about getting some actual hands-on CPR practice?

In almost every community the local offices of the American Heart Association and the American National Red Cross sponsor regular CPR classes. The standard Heart Association course usually takes four to six hours to complete; the Red Cross course, ten to twelve hours.

But there is good news for those readers who, having learned most of the factual material presented in this book, may not need such lengthy instruction. Both the Red Cross and Heart Association are adding new modular, self-paced CPR courses, where you work at your own speed, checking in with an instructor or supervisor when you're ready to demonstrate your mastery of a given skill.

Those who have read this book should be able to complete one of these self-paced courses very quickly and easily.

Of the two programs, the Red Cross course may be the easier and faster route for readers of this book, for it allows those with previous knowledge or training to demonstrate that background quickly and then get on to mannikin practice. But with this book as background, you'll have no trouble with either course.

How long should you expect to take to complete these courses? That will vary among individuals (and also according to how well the course is organized, the number of mannikins and instructors available, how well students' time is used, and other variables), but you should be able to finish in less than half the time required by most students—perhaps as little as two to three hours, in just one session.

If there is no Red Cross or Heart Association chapter in your city, call the local emergency medical service, police or fire department, or city or county health department for information on CPR classes in your area.

Upon successful completion of one of these authorized programs, you'll earn a card attesting to your certification to perform CPR in emergencies.

This card is valuable in two ways: first, because it may help gain for you the protection of your state's "Good Samaritan" laws, to protect you from a lawsuit over your use of CPR.*

And second, it also serves as your admission ticket to periodic "refresher" and "update" CPR classes. These subsequent recertification classes are extremely important, for they not only polish your skills—all of us get rusty at psychomotor skills after a while—but also allow you to learn of new methods and new techniques to make you an even more effective rescuer.

You won't want to miss a chance to take a recertification class every year or two.

One last note on teaching and learning CPR: After you've mastered the skill and gotten your certification card, you're going to be eager for your friends to learn CPR.

For one thing, they're your best chance of survival in the event *you* suffer a heart attack or other emergency involving breathing and circulation.

But for another, you'll find once you know CPR that it's a great feeling: that sure knowledge that in an emergency you'll know what to do, how to save a life. You'll know that you'll never suffer that awful feeling of helplessness most people endure when they come upon an accident or other medical emergency. You'll know that in most serious cases you'll never have to simply stand by, just watching—perhaps watching as someone dies, needlessly—because no one knew what to do to help.

---

*More on Good Samaritan laws in Chapter 13.

You'll *know*.

And that's a very satisfying feeling, one you'll be eager to share with those close to you.

But please, once you know CPR, don't try to teach your friends how to do it. Just as you needed the background information found in this book and understanding of how to detect heart attacks, plus mannikin-practice time, they'll also need those facts, that experience, to become skilled, self-confident rescuers.

There's more in Chapter 15 on how to encourage others to learn CPR. For now, just remember: *Never, never attempt to teach someone yourself.*

5 What happens when a heart stops

You needn't become an expert on cardiopulmonary physiology in order to perform CPR well and save a life.

But knowing a little about how the heart, lungs, and brain work together, and just what happens when that event we call a "heart attack" occurs, will help you better understand how and why CPR works so well.

As we breathe, we draw in fresh air containing about 21 percent oxygen and just a trace of carbon dioxide. That air passes in through our mouth and nose, down the windpipe, and out through the bronchial tubes into our lungs. In the lungs, a marvelous and complex exchange process takes place: The lungs extract that oxygen from the air, put it into our blood, and draw from the blood the gas, carbon dioxide, that our body creates as waste.

The carbon dioxide is discarded as we exhale. In fact, air

exiting our lungs is down to only about 16 percent oxygen but has picked up 4 percent carbon dioxide.

As our lungs extract the oxygen from the air we breathe and get it into our blood, the heart is pumping that blood throughout the body, bringing this fresh supply of oxygen to every bit of tissue in the body.

It is this oxygen, carried by the blood, pumped by the heart, which is the "staff of life" for our bodies: tissue must have oxygen to live.

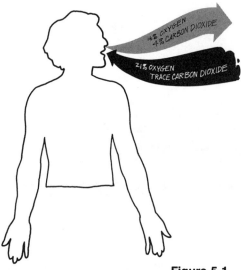

Figure 5-1

The brain, acting as the body's control center, is exceptionally greedy about this oxygen. It demands a generous, uninterrupted supply. Indeed, brain tissue requires perhaps ten times as much oxygen as other tissue; our brains use up a fourth of all the oxygen we consume.

If the brain, or control center, dies, all other functions cease as well. Because it is irreversible, brain death means certain death for the entire human body.

So in a very real sense, CPR isn't for keeping the heart or lungs alive but for keeping the *brain* alive, through providing that supply of fresh oxygen when our hearts and lungs are not up to the task.

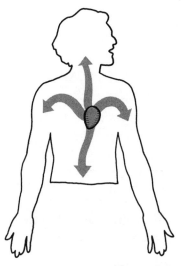

Figure 5-2

Brain death has become the new measure of whether a person is alive or dead. Once, it all seemed so simple: If a person had neither heartbeat nor respiration—no pulse, no breathing—he was dead.

But today we know better.

For researchers have learned there is a period of four to six minutes after the heart has stopped pumping freshly oxygenated blood through the body when there is still enough residual oxygen in the brain to keep it alive.

And this has led to two new definitions of death:

clinical death, that point at which breathing and heartbeat have ceased; and

biological death, that point four to six minutes later when the brain has begun, irreversibly, to die.

These definitions are important for the CPR rescuer, for they give us the key to how and why CPR works and show us how quickly we must work in order to capture that life before it slips away.

The graph in Figure 5-3 illustrates how rapidly our chances of saving a victim fall as time passes.

In CPR, our task is to intervene in that deadly curve as soon as possible after the heart attack, and thereby to stabilize the victim

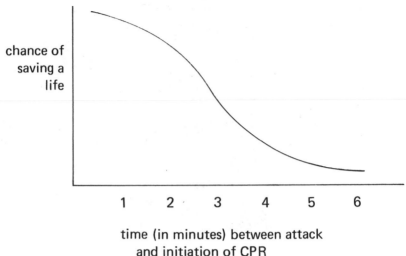

chance of
saving a
life

1   2   3   4   5   6

time (in minutes) between attack
and initiation of CPR

Figure 5-3

with our artificial respiration and artificial circulation until his heart can be restarted.

When paramedics arrive they may replace your mouth-to-mouth breathing with a "breathing bag"-type respirator or an automatic-feed oxygen mask and tank. They may apply a sharp electrical shock to the victim's chest, using defibrillation paddles, to jolt the heart back into action. They may administer a drug, such as Lydocaine, to stimulate the heart and promote a steady beat.

All of these steps can help restart a failed heart, revive a victim otherwise destined to die. But they cannot work if brain death has occurred: There simply is no patient, no life, to bring back.

Once we begin CPR, we no longer have the benefit of that curve shown in Figure 5-3, that four-to-six minute period during which a victim can live without CPR. At its best, CPR only provides about one-third the cardiac output of a normal, healthy heart at work on its own. Thus with CPR we are merely stabilizing the victim, maintaining him or her in a holding pattern with a low but life-sustaining level of cardiac pumping until more sophisticated care, such as electronic defibrillation, is available.

Before we continue, let us clear up one point of terminology.

The phrase *heart attack*, used throughout this book, is medically inexact. Some physicians use the term *coronary event* in its place, to indicate that there are several kinds of heart attacks, or coronary events, which can stop the heart and kill. To avoid repeated use of such complex and often intimidating terms as myocardial infarction, ventricular fibrillation, ventricular tachycardia, atrial fibrillation and others, we will continue to refer to those incidents when the heart stops as heart attacks.

For our purposes, a heart attack is an incident in which the heart stops beating, there is no pulse or breathing, and the victim is clinically dead.

It is at that point that we go to work to save his life, using what we call "the ABCs of CPR."

6 Detecting a heart attack

The best way to do CPR may be never to do it at all . . . because you are so alert to the symptoms of an impending heart attack, in yourself or another, that you're able to summon help or get the victim to emergency facilities before the heart attack happens.

A victim's chances of surviving a heart attack are many times greater if it occurs in an emergency room or in an ambulance than if it hits when he is away from professional help. Indeed, complex care systems can often forestall the heart attack altogether—if the victim is in the hands of medical professionals before the attack occurs.

Although some persons collapse from heart attacks without any apparent warning, most cardiac arrests are preceded by one or more of several easily learned, easily detected symptoms. The first step in becoming a competent CPR rescuer is knowing these early-warning signs, and knowing when and how to act on them.

23

For many persons the first sign of a heart attack is a terrible, terrifying pain in the chest. It is often described by survivors as "crushing," "the worst pain I've ever felt in my life." Some victims say it was "like an elephant standing on my chest."

Oddly, other victims describe the feeling not so much in terms of pain but as tightness, pressure, or "fullness": "It was like my chest was in a huge vise"; "I just felt like I was going to blow up, like my chest was going to explode"; "I thought it was just bad 'gas' pains."

Ah, the killer phrase: "It must be gas."   ·

Those four words may be the most dangerous in the English language, for they may have killed more people than any others. If you feel what you think may be gas pains, and they do not quickly go away, you may be in the early stages of having a heart attack.

So the first key sign of a heart attack in most victims is

a *pain, pressure or squeezing in the chest* which does not go away or lessen.

The second sign—and a critical confirmation of the true meaning of what you may have thought were only gas pains—is a second pain, anywhere above the waist.

This second pain very commonly appears in the underside of the upper arm, usually on the victim's left side. Or it may appear in the jaw, on the right side of the chest, or elsewhere. Sometimes it seems to radiate outward toward the heart; other times it seems to be a separate pain, unconnected to the chest discomfort.

Thus, our second warning sign is

a second pain *anywhere above the waist.*

If you or someone near you feels a chest pain or pressure, squeezing, or fullness in the chest, and it is joined by a second pain above the waist, act immediately. Do not wait for other symptoms to appear. You may never notice them; you may be unconscious before you can act on them.

Call for help immediately.

The other common warning signs of an impending heart attack are sweating, nausea, shortness of breath, and an overall feeling of weakness, of suddenly being very tired.

Remember that you don't have to have all these symptoms to suffer a heart attack. This isn't a laundry list, on which you must check off every item. Act on the first two primary warning signs. And act quickly!

People often act stupidly when they fear they may be having a heart attack. Psychologists tell us these "denial behaviors" or "avoidance behaviors" reflect our deep-seated fears of our own mortality. It can't be happening to us. It's always the other guy who has heart attacks, not you or me.

Figure 6-1

If you think you're having a heart attack . . .

√ REVIEW the symptoms: Pain in the chest? A second pain? Sweating? Nausea? Dizziness?

√ If you have two or more symptoms, ACT NOW!

√ If alone, CALL your local emergency medical service.

√ If with others, ASK SOMEONE TO CALL the emergency service for you.

√ ASK SOMEONE TO STAY with you.

√ SIT or LIE DOWN.

√ Try to REMAIN CALM.

Fill in these numbers now:

Emergency Medical Service serving your home

_____

Emergency Medical Service serving your office

_____

Remember the first sentence of this book? Remember your odds—everyone's odds—of dying of heart disease?

It may be you this time.

Act in a way that can help save your life, not virtually assure your death.

In an office or institutional setting, one of the most common reactions for the heart attack victim is to leave his or her desk and walk to the nearest restroom. Not, mind you, to approach a friend or co-worker, mention the symptoms, and ask for help—or even a reassuring word. No, the victim slips off to the restroom, unnoticed.

He or she enters a stall, sits down on the toilet—fully clothed—and begins hoping the symptoms will go away. The next thing anyone knows is when someone enters the restroom a few minutes later and finds our victim's body slumped onto the floor, feet sticking out under the stall door—dead.

If you think you're having a heart attack or if you think someone around you may be about to have one, don't let these foolish denial behaviors kill you or them!

If you start experiencing the symptoms, go to someone, ask her to call for an ambulance, and stay with her. Ideally that should be someone who knows CPR, but even if not, at least she can telephone for assistance. You can hardly do that for yourself if you collapse, unconscious.

If someone near you begins to show or speak of any of the warning signs, ask him how he feels. Make a quick survey of his symptoms: Ask if he has chest pains; if there is a pain in his arm, jaw, or elsewhere; if he feels nauseous or dizzy. Make him focus on you and answer your questions. Often a victim will act dazed and will simply stare back, not answering. By asking specific questions, rather than general, "how do you feel?" inquiries, you can make him pay attention to you.

If he wants to sit or lie down, by all means help him to do so.

And if you're convinced he has one or more of the warning signs of a heart attack, send someone else to call for an ambulance, or take the victim with you to the nearest telephone, and make that call yourself. Don't frighten the victim unnecessarily; but don't take "no" for an answer, either.

If you believe you are having a heart attack, and you ask someone else to call for help for you, accompany her to the telephone. If you are calling for someone else, try to get him to walk to the telephone with you; or at least keep him within sight as you make the call.

Never leave a possible heart attack victim alone, even for a few seconds: If he or she collapses, you must be able to begin CPR at once.

Too often a couple will be comfortably ensconced at home in the evening, perhaps watching television. The husband complains of chest pains, perhaps a second pain, and sensing their seriousness, asks his wife to drive him to the hospital. Unwilling to be seen by emergency room personnel in the tattered old housedress or gown she's wearing, she ducks into the bedroom for a moment to change and run a brush through her hair.

When she returns she finds her husband slumped on the

Figure 6-2

If you are with someone
you think may be having a heart attack . . .

✓Allow him to SIT or LIE DOWN, if he wishes.

✓TALK TO HIM; make him focus on you. Ask for specific symptoms: pain in the chest, second pain, sweating, nausea, dizziness.

✓If he has two or more symptoms, ACT NOW!

✓CALL the local emergency medical service.

✓STAY WITH THE VICTIM. If possible, ask him to walk with you to the telephone when you call for help, or use a telephone in the room where he is sitting or lying down.

✓WATCH THE VICTIM closely. If he slips into unconsciousness, begin the ABCs of CPR at once.

✓REMAIN CALM. Remember: the victim's life may rest in your hands. Focus on your CPR training. Repeat the ABCs aloud as you work, if that helps you concentrate.

floor: The heart attack has already happened, and valuable seconds have been lost.

Never worry about vanity in getting help for yourself or another. Emergency room crews have seen people in far worse clothes, far worse shape than you; they won't notice the old shirt, the torn gown, the slippers, and the hair rollers.

Never leave a likely heart attack victim—even for a second!

When we interview those few persons who survive hiding in a toilet stall or refusing to allow their friends to call an ambulance until they actually collapse, we hear the most bizarre explanations:

> Well, you know, I just thought it was gas, and I didn't want to call the ambulance and everything . . . all those flashing lights and sirens, the guys in the funny white suits. What if it had just been gas?

What if it *hadn't* been a heart attack?

So what if it hadn't?

The victim would have had a fast ride to the nearest emergency room, while being closely observed by paramedics especially trained to offer emergency assistance. At the hospital he would have been examined, connected to an electrocardiograph, prepared for defibrillation, if needed, interviewed by a staff doctor, perhaps by a cardiologist.

He would have been watched closely for an hour or two or three, then—if it was certain that the pain was only muscular, or perhaps even from gas—allowed to return home.

The potential victim and those around him—co-workers, friends, family—would have known that all was well, that in that first frightening hour after the onset of possible heart attack symptoms the person they knew and loved and cared about was getting the best possible care and attention. And in the event that the worst came to pass—that it was a heart attack in progress—they'd have known he was in the best hands, in the best possible situation to survive the attack.

That's *bad*?

Never be afraid to call for an ambulance because you're not absolutely sure the symptoms presage a heart attack. Unless you have an M.D. tacked onto your name, you're not competent to make that decision.

You *are* competent to consider the sudden appearance of the warning signs that commonly precede heart attacks, and when they are in evidence, to seek medical help at once.

Do not let a life be lost because you were uncertain and indecisive, nor because a victim argues against your seeking help.

Get help. *Fast.*

7 Getting help

Quick: How do you call for an ambulance in your community?

Dial 0 and let the operator handle it?

Well maybe, in some kinds of emergencies, but have you dialed 0 lately? Remember how long it took to get an answer? And all an operator can do is take down the information, call the right number him- or herself, and pass on your request. (And the training and good intentions of telephone company operators notwithstanding, whenever information is relayed through a third party there is the possibility of a mistake in translation: "Was that 2813 17th Avenue? Or 2318 7th Avenue? Or . . .")

Call the police? Probably not, unless your community has a police-dispatched ambulance operation. And in any case, do you know the police department's emergency number? In a cardiac emergency there's no time to look up telephone numbers.

Call the fire department? That's OK if they dispatch ambulances in your community, but again, that's unlikely. And do you know *their* number?

Stop right now and take a look at the inside front cover of your telephone directory. Find the emergency medical services number for your neighborhood and *memorize it*. Then find the number to call from your office, school, or other place you spend your days. *Memorize it, too.*

There will be no test at the end of this chapter; but there may well come someday, without warning or chance for review, a real-life test, when you will need to dial for an ambulance or tell someone else how to—without time to fumble with a telephone directory, look up a number, or relay the information through an operator.

In many communities—more than 800 by the beginning of 1978—there is a single emergency number, through which a citizen can summon a policeman, a fireman, or an ambulance.

That number is 911.

The idea originated in England, which has had a single, three-digit emergency number, 999, since the 1930s. It was immensely helpful during World War II, when authorities credited the existence of centralized emergency services dispatching centers with saving thousands of lives following German air raids.

The system has worked even better during peacetime. Adjusted for population figures, four times as many Americans as Britons die from fires—because the British can summon firemen so much more quickly and efficiently. And although there are no hard figures on how many lives are saved in England through increased efficiency in summoning ambulances, all concede the number is very large.

If your community has 911 emergency service, memorize that number, teach it to your kids, co-workers, spouse, and friends. And be thankful you live in an area so blessed.

If your area *doesn't* have 911 service, find out why not.

Both Bell and independent telephone companies have been generally cooperative about installing 911 service since the first 911 system was set up in Haleyville, Alabama, in the early 1960s. In most cases the emergency number can be dialed even from pay phones without coins—an important consideration if you don't have two dimes in your pocket.

But someone has to demand the service. Talk with your local elected officials: selectmen, mayor, commissioners, police chief, sheriff, fire inspector, the people who need to know how much you want this service.

Make enough noise, in the right places, and your community will get 911 service.

Knowing the correct telephone number to dial isn't all there is to summoning emergency assistance.

You'll need to give the dispatcher the correct address, your estimate of the urgency of the situation, perhaps the telephone number you're calling from, possibly the nearest major intersection. And you'll have to do that quickly, intelligibly, without needless chatter or elaboration.

You'll also need to remember to stay on the line until you're told to hang up.

The simple rule: When you call for help, stay as calm as the situation permits, answer questions quickly and simply, and don't hang up until you're told to do so.

To a person, emergency medical services dispatchers tell a universal horror story. For some, it happens every week, even every day. They answer the emergency line and an anguished caller spurts out

"Help! Come quick! I need an ambulance! My wife . . . I think it's a heart attack. Hurry up! My God, I think she's dying!"

BANG! The receiver slams down.

And the dispatcher, caught up in the horror of the moment, sits there and weeps.

For he or she knows that somewhere out in that city, a man is kneeling next to his wife, desperate, frightened, praying that she will survive—and confident that help is on the way.

Except that it isn't.

Because they don't know where to send the ambulance.

He hung up before giving an address.

Practice this little drill with your family. Use two telephones (or two shoes, two sticks, two anythings) to make it more realistic. Let one person play the "caller," the other, the "dispatcher."

The caller explains help is needed, gives the address, then briefly explains the nature of the emergency.

The dispatcher asks the caller to repeat the address. He may also ask for the caller's telephone number or a nearby cross street (to help the driver find the address quickly). He may ask if the victim is in a multistory building and if so, on what floor and in what office or apartment number he can be found. If it is evening, he may ask that the lights be turned on, the front door left wide open. He may ask if someone else there can be sent out to the curb, perhaps to that nearby intersection, to flag down the driver and direct him to the right house.

To each question the caller responds quickly and succinctly, without unnecessary chatter or elaboration.

Finally the dispatcher tells the caller to hang up and go back to the victim's aid.

A little role playing of that kind can make an effective caller of even an eight- or ten-year-old child. And several runthroughs will reassure an adult that in an emergency he or she will know what to do, how to summon help most quickly.

If you live or work in a highrise apartment or office building, think now about what you'd do in case of an emergency.

If you're with someone who collapses from an apparent heart attack, above the ground floor, and there are others on the scene who can help, this is the sequence:

1. Tell someone to call for an ambulance, and if necessary, tell him or her the telephone number.
2. Tell two others to ride downstairs in the elevator together. One holds the elevator at the first floor for the immediate (and exclusive) use of the ambulance crew, while the other goes to the front door to guide the paramedics, upon their arrival, directly to the elevator.
3. Meanwhile, you begin CPR to keep the victim alive until the paramedics arrive.

A family (or office) drill on this routine is helpful, too, and can save precious minutes in an emergency.

Sometimes it makes more sense to take a potential heart attack victim to a hospital yourself, rather than calling and waiting for an ambulance.

If, for example, you're on a hunting trip in the woods, and a fellow hunter begins suffering chest pains, it would probably be far faster to walk him slowly to a car and then drive directly to the nearest hospital than to hike out to a telephone, call for an ambulance, and wait while the paramedics searched for you in the woods.

Or if you live in a rural area, and your spouse begins to display the critical warning signs of an oncoming heart attack, you could probably make it to a hospital in half the time it would take for an ambulance to come out from town and then return with him or her to that same hospital.

But if the victim actually does suffer the attack on the way, you must be prepared to stop immediately and begin CPR. You cannot continue on to the hospital, hoping you'll make it in time. Roadside CPR will be necessary.

Effective CPR must be begun *at once* for a victim who lapses into unconsciousness.

You'll also want to know where to take the victim.

You can't keep up with the location and capabilities of every hospital in your state, but you should make inquiries *now* to learn the locations of hospitals in your immediate area which maintain twenty-four-hour emergency-care facilities. Do not simply assume that all hospitals maintain proper emergency rooms; many no longer do, and even among those offering emergency care, a surprising number do not offer adequate care for the coronary victim.

Ask your doctor where *he* would prefer to be taken if he suffered a heart attack. Ask about alternatives, in the event that you are with, or come across, a coronary victim at some distance from that hospital.

By getting this information now and deciding to which local hospital you would take a victim you must transport, you'll save fumbling, indecision, and delays when you need to move quickly.

8 Learning the ABCs

The steps in performing CPR are easy to learn, and a simple memory trick makes them easy to remember in emergencies.

That trick lies in the names of the three steps:

A, *or airway*
B, *or breathing*
C, *or circulation*

These simple names tell us which of the victim's needs must be dealt with, and in what order, to save his life. And when you've learned CPR this way, the "ABCs of CPR" routine will always be there when you need it, so that you won't have to fumble around in a crisis, trying to remember what comes next.

Because we deal with *every* emergency in which CPR can help by using these same steps, in the same order, there are no

special exceptions or alternative sequences to learn and remember. Once you've got the ABCs mastered, you've mastered
CPR.

The first step, *A*, or *airway*, is simply a matter of opening the
victim's airway—a path from nose and mouth through the
windpipe and into the lungs—so that breathing becomes possible.

The second step, *B*, or *breathing*, involves checking to see if
the victim is breathing, and if he is not, breathing for him.

And *C*, or *circulation*, requires checking for a pulse, to see if
his heart is beating on its own; if it is not, we provide an artificial
heartbeat by pressing on his chest with our hands.

Simple, isn't it?

We'll take those steps one at a time. However, remember,
although they are simply and easily learned, each requires practice to achieve sufficient skill to save a life, and that practice must
be on a mannikin, not another person.

AIRWAY

In any collapse—even so simple and seemingly unthreatening an
event as passing out and falling down—the back of the tongue can
slump down, blocking the windpipe. If this is not corrected
quickly, no oxygen can get through to the lungs; there is no fresh
supply of oxygen for the brain; and the brain—and our victim—
can die.

So our first step in performing CPR is *opening the airway*.
And it's quick and easy to do.

With the victim on his back, on the ground or floor or other
firm, horizontal support,* quickly kneel next to him, opposite his
shoulder. With one hand on each shoulder, give him a gentle
shake (as you would to awaken a heavy sleeper) and shout "Are
you OK? Are you all right?"

---

*Never try to perform CPR on someone on a bed or other soft, springy
support (such as a sofa). If chest compressions become necessary, you will find it
impossible to actually compress the victim's chest: You will simply be bouncing
him up and down on the bedsprings. The floor is the best, easiest, most reliable
support for a victim.

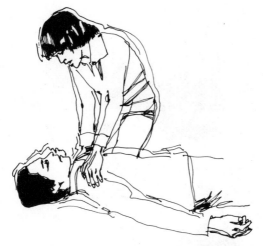

Figure 8-1

This is important: Before we begin trying to rescue someone, we want to make absolutely sure they really need our help. If you come upon someone lying in the grass, you don't want to begin a full rescue only to discover he's taking a sunbath!

If there is no response, slip your hand *nearest his feet* under his neck, and simultaneously place your other hand flat on his forehead. With one motion, pull up under his neck and press down on his forehead.

You've just completed step A—opening the airway.

Easy, wasn't it?

Strange as it seems, opening the airway is often all it takes to save a life. The victim may cough, sputter, gasp, or wheeze a little, then resume normal, if somewhat labored, breathing. If he does, fine: You've just saved his life. If not, you need to go on to the *B* step.

Remember: Not every rescue requires all three (A, B, C) steps. Often only A, or only A and B, are needed.

BREATHING

Our next job is to determine if, once we opened his airway, the victim has begun to breathe again on his own. And if he has not, we must breathe for him, to get that vital oxygen into his lungs.

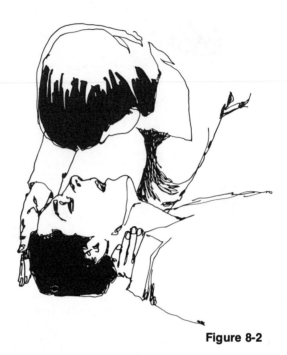

Figure 8-2

We use three simultaneous checks to learn whether he has begun to breathe again. All three are performed in the same position, without moving our hands or knees from the "open the airway" position.

Lean forward over the victim, holding your head close to his, your face turned 90 degrees toward his feet. Your head should be positioned just an inch or so above his face, and your ear should be directly above his nose.

In that position, we make the three tests: *looking*, *listening*, and *feeling* for breathing.

Looking is simple: With your head turned toward the victim's feet, sight across his chest and watch for the rise and fall of the chest, indicating breathing.

Listening is easy, too: Just listen for air exhaled from his nose.

And *feeling* is the easiest of all: With your ear over his nose, your cheek falls naturally just over his mouth, so you can feel air exhaled from his lungs through the mouth.

All three tests are done simultaneously, and they shouldn't take more than a few seconds.

40

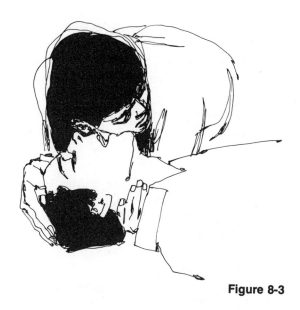

Figure 8-3

Because the circumstances surrounding the accident or attack can make it difficult to determine the presence or absence of breathing via one or another of these tests alone, *we always use all three.*

Skeptical that all three are really needed?

You could always *see* someone's chest rise and fall, right? What if you're aiding a heart attack victim who has collapsed at a football game on a cold November day? She's wearing long underwear, two shirts, three sweaters, and a bulky down parka. With three or four inches of clothing covering her chest, do you really think you'd be able to see her chest rise and fall?

But you could always *hear* her breathing, right? Especially with your ear just an inch from her nose? Supposing 70,000 fans jump up, screaming, cheering for a long pass completion. Still think you could hear that gentle wheeze of exhaled air?

But *feeling*—there's the best test. Because even if we can't see or hear breathing, by looking and listening, we can almost always detect the presence of breathing through *feeling* it on our cheek.

Still skeptical? Try this: Hold your hand up in front of your face, fingers outstretched, palm just an inch or so from your mouth. Now exhale very, very gently a time or two. Feel that warm, moist stuff on your hand?

That's the moisture carried by your breath, and it's concrete evidence of the presence of breathing. Breath *feels* warm and damp.

And by using all three tests, you'll be confident that you *know*, not just suspect, whether or not a victim is breathing on his own.

If, airway opened, our victim has begun to breathe on his own, we have already saved his life. Opening the airway was all that was needed. Keep the airway open—your hands and knees should not have moved from their original positions—until other help arrives, to make sure the victim can continue to breathe until he fully regains consciousness.

If there is no spontaneous breathing, we go on to the second half of B: giving the victim some air.

And we do that through mouth-to-mouth breathing, or *artificial respiration*. Like the rest of CPR, it's easier than it sounds and takes far longer to describe than to use in a real rescue.

Figure 8-4

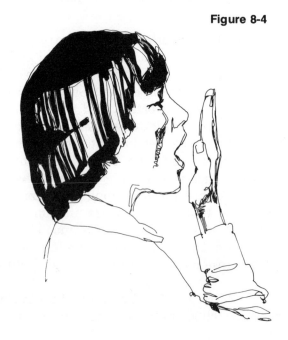

With your hands still in the "open the airway" position, reach over with the thumb and forefinger of the hand atop the victim's forehead and pinch the bottom of his nose shut.

Open your mouth wide and seal your lips over his. Give him four big, full breaths—each at least twice the volume of your normal breaths. Of course, you'll have to lift your head up an inch or so between breaths in order to refill your lungs, then reseal your lips over his as you deliver that breath. Otherwise, there should be no delay here: Get those breaths into him as fast as you can.

Between breaths, as you're refilling your lungs, look quickly again toward his feet, to see that his chest is falling. As you are refilling your own lungs, his chest will be falling as he "exhales" the breath you've blown into him.

If when you blow into the victim the air does not seem to get through—if it's like trying to exhale with a hand sealed over your mouth—you probably haven't lifted his neck enough in opening his airway. Reposition his head, lifting harder under the neck and pressing down a bit more on his forehead. Try the breaths again and you'll probably find they go in just fine this time.

When you've given those four breaths, you've completed the entire B step.

Just three simple actions—opening the airway, checking for breathing, and giving four big breaths, if needed—and you're

Figure 8-5

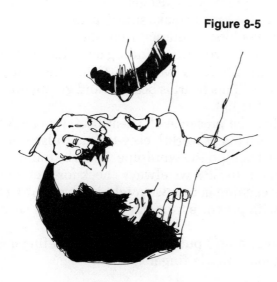

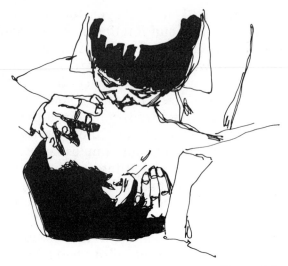

Figure 8-6

two-thirds of the way through already! This is probably going to be a lot easier than you thought.

CIRCULATION

If the victim has suffered a heart attack—if his heart has come to a stop, and he is pulseless—just getting that air into his lungs isn't enough. You also have to make sure that air gets from the lungs up to his brain, via blood pumped from the heart.

Just as B had two parts—finding out if he was breathing, and giving him breath if he was not—C has the same two steps: checking to see if his heart is beating, and giving him an artificial heartbeat if it is not.

To detect the presence of a heartbeat, we check the victim's *carotid pulse*. This powerful, easy-to-find pulse lies in the neck, tucked in just behind the windpipe. It can be found on both sides of the neck, but in CPR we always check for it on our side of the victim. (In reaching across we might inadvertently choke off the windpipe with pressure from our fingers as they searched for the pulse.)

To find a carotid pulse first make a "two-finger salute" with your index and middle fingers.

44

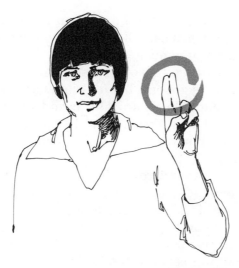

Figure 8-7

Imagine a dotted line drawn down the middle of the front of your neck. Place your two fingertips astride this line, and slide them down to the Adam's apple. At that point, slide your fingers off the line and down a little on the side of the neck until they slip into the narrow groove which runs up and down the neck. (For the technical-minded, this is the gap between the heavy strap muscles of the neck and the windpipe.)

Figure 8-8

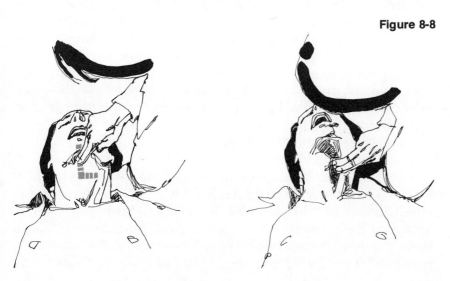

The carotid artery, and thus the carotid pulse, lies right in that groove. Apply just a bit of pressure with your fingertips and you'll feel it thumping away.

If you've just tried this on yourself without finding a pulse, don't worry: You've got one, but it's often hard to find your own. Try it with a friend. Make sure your friend's head is tilted backwards, as it would be in a real rescue. And don't grope around up near the jawline: You can find a pulse there, but it's not the one we're looking for.

When you've found your friend's carotid pulse, find someone else's. Then another and another and another still. Practice finding the carotid pulses of as many cooperative friends as you can, for your self-confidence in your ability to find a pulse is very important: You must be able to locate pulses reliably, so that if you check a victim and seem to find no pulse, you're sure there is none.

Though there is never time to be wasted in a CPR rescue, checking for a victim's pulse is one point where we do take a few extra seconds to make certain our diagnosis of pulselessness is correct. *Take as much as ten or fifteen seconds* to make absolutely sure a victim has no pulse before proceeding with the rescue.

In practicing CPR, or performing it in a real emergency, most rescuers keep their hand on the victim's forehead in place—just as it has been since the beginning of the rescue—and use the hand that has been supporting the neck to make the two-finger salute and check for the carotid pulse. But if your victim is elderly or has a pudgy neck, it may be easier to find the pulse by keeping that hand in place under the neck, to keep the fatty folds of the neck pulled taut, while the hand formerly atop the forehead is used to check for the pulse.

Use the position that works best for you.

If there is a pulse, you will not need to give the victim an artificial heartbeat by compressing his chest—he already has circulation—but you may need to continue breathing for him. Return to the open-airway position, check for breathing, and if there is none, give one breath every five seconds. An easy way to count and time these breaths is to say to yourself, "One thousand

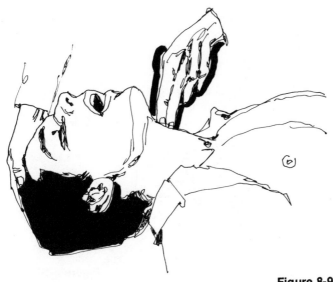

Figure 8-9

and ONE, one thousand and TWO, one thousand and THREE, one thousand and FOUR, BREATHE! One thousand and ONE, one thousand. . . ." (The BREATHE! would be inaudible, of course, for you would on that count be breathing into the victim.)

If there is no pulse, the victim needs chest compressions to pump throughout his body that freshly oxygenated blood you have helped create by breathing for him.

To do chest compressions properly, we need to understand a little of the anatomy of the chest.

Contrary to what you may have heard about the heart lying way over on the left side of the chest, it actually lies very near the center, directly beneath the sternum, or centerplate of the rib cage. The sternum is in some ways like a big hinge, holding the ribs together in front and allowing a certain amount of flexion. It is because of this flexion that CPR can pump blood for a victim whose heart is not beating: We press down on the sternum, squeezing the heart between it and the backbone, thus forcing blood out just as if the heart were beating on its own.

However, connected to the bottom of the sternum is a little bony protrusion, known as the xiphoid process. Unfortunately, it is rather poorly connected to the sternum itself, and pressure over

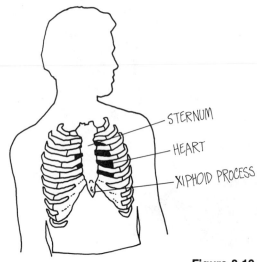

STERNUM

HEART

XIPHOID PROCESS

Figure 8-10

the xiphoid can break it off, sending it plunging into the lungs, liver, spleen, and other internal organs, like a tiny arrowhead loose within the victim's chest.

So in order to do safe, effective chest compressions, we must learn to place our hands—*accurately and consistently*—in the correct place atop the sternum, just a little higher than the xiphoid.

Figure 8-11

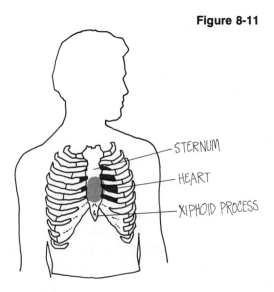

STERNUM

HEART

XIPHOID PROCESS

And we use the xiphoid itself as our landmark to guide us to that correct position.

To better understand the parts of the chest, take off your shirt or blouse, and underwear and locate some of these anatomical structures in your own chest.

Place your hands at your sides and, pressing inward, bring them up to the bottom of the rib cage. It will be the first hard, resistant area above your wait.

Now follow the curve of that bottom rib up and toward the center of your chest. Notice as you move along that the bottom of your rib cage forms an inverted V with the point of the V aiming straight up.

The xiphoid lies right at the top of that V, at that point where the ribs come together.

Now make a two-finger salute again, and place those two fingers at the top of an imaginary line drawn down the middle of your chest.

Slide the two fingers down toward your waist, exerting a little pressure, until they "fall off" as they pass beyond the xiphoid process into the area of the stomach.

Follow the sketches in this chapter as you do these exercises. As you feel your chest, identify and name the structures you're touching—bottom rib, sternum, xiphoid process.

Figure 8-12

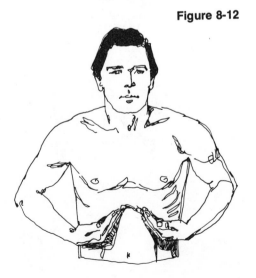

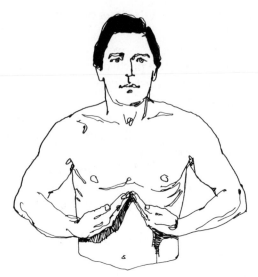

Figure 8-13

Figure 8-14

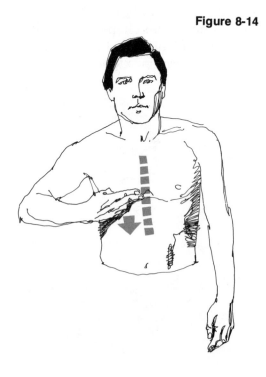

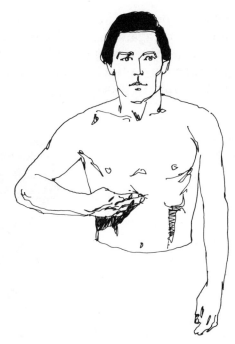

Figure 8-15

When you've got a pretty good idea how chests are put together, you're ready to learn how to compress the chest of a heart attack victim to give him or her an artificial heartbeat.

But remember: *Never, never practice compressing the chest of someone who does not need CPR!* You may wish to practice locating your hands ONLY on the chest of a friend, but all actual chest-compression practice must be done on a special training mannikin.*

---

*The reasons for avoiding chest-compression practice on someone who does not need CPR are simple. First, until you are skilled in the task, through mannikin practice, there is a danger of pressing too hard or in the wrong place, perhaps breaking a rib or breaking off the xiphoid—both of which could cause very serious internal injuries. Second, and even more importantly, a beating heart has its own rhythm, and superimposing your own compression rhythm over that natural rhythm can confuse the heart muscle, causing it to stop beating or to move into what physicians call *ventricular fibrillation:* a rapid fluttering motion which does not move blood.

Thus, chest-compression practice on someone whose heart is already beating on its own could seriously injure or kill him.

Never practice on a living person, always on mannikins!

51

To locate the correct position for chest compressions, make that two-finger salute once again, using the index and middle fingers of your hand *nearer the victim's feet.** Place those fingers on that imaginary centerline on the chest, and slide them down until they are atop the xiphoid process.

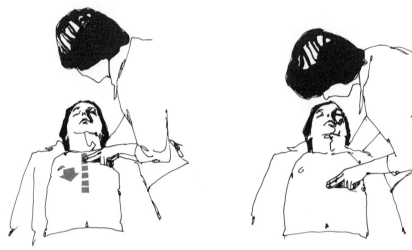

Figure 8-16

Keeping those two fingers in place, place the heel of your other hand immediately next to them, higher on the chest.

You have used those two fingers, in effect, as a measuring jig, just as a carpenter uses a little jig to position a board or tool correctly. Those two fingers, placed atop the xiphoid, are your personal measuring tools to make certain you will compress the chest in the proper place.

---

*You've probably been wondering about all these instructions calling for the use of "the hand nearer the victim's feet." Why not just say "the left hand" or "the right hand"?

Competent rescuers should be able to perform CPR from both sides of a collapsed victim. Learning hand-placement by using left-and-right rules confuses the rescuer when he moves to the opposite side of a victim; everything seems backward.

Do not let yourself fall into the habit of thinking "this is always done with the left hand" and "this is done with the right." Remember the relationship of your hands to the victim's body, and you'll find CPR comfortable and natural from both sides of a victim.

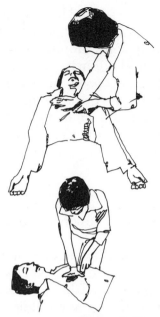

Figure 8-17

Figure 8-18

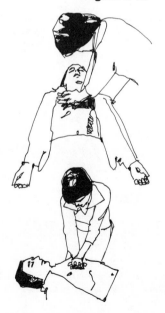

When the heel of your second hand is firmly in place, lift the two-finger-salute hand, place it atop the other, and clasp your fingers together. The top hand should pry your fingers up a little, so that only the *heel* of the bottom hand actually touches the chest.

With your hands in this position, begin chest compressions, pressing down, pausing an instant, coming up to completely release pressure (but not lose contact with the chest) for another instant, then compressing again. Keep your elbows in, your arms straight as you compress, and let your back and shoulder muscles do the work.

We compress a victim's chest at a rate of *eighty times a minute*—a little faster than once per second.

And we press the chest downward from 1½ to 2 inches per stroke.

As you compress, make certain there is a tiny pause at the top and bottom of each stroke. And avoid sharp "stabbing" compressions, which do little good since they cannot move blood from the heart; also avoid "bouncing" around, thereby losing position on the chest. Your bottom hand never leaves the victim's chest but completely releases pressure between compressions.

Figure 8-19

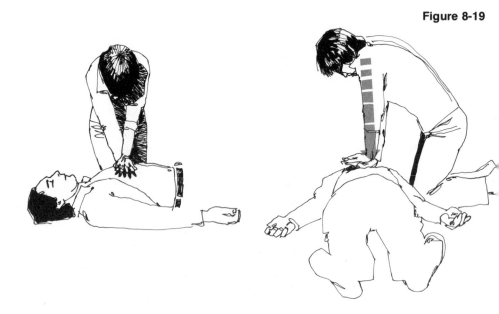

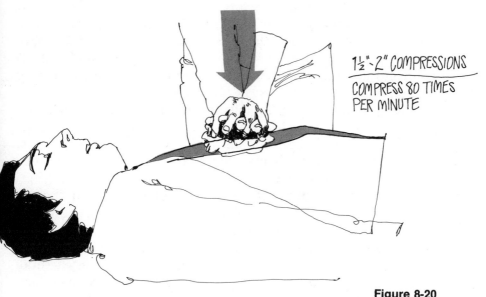

1½"-2" COMPRESSIONS
COMPRESS 80 TIMES
PER MINUTE

Figure 8-20

Before we go any further it will be helpful to get a good idea of just how fast an 80-compressions-per-minute rate feels and to get a clear sense of just what a 1½-to-2-inch stroke involves.

If you have a musician's metronome handy, you're in luck: Set it at 80 beats per minute and count along with it as it ticks away. Most rescuers find it best to learn to count "ONE and TWO and THREE and . . . FOURTEEN and FIFTEEN," both to keep up with their compressison count and to help maintain the right rhythm.

If you don't have (and can't borrow) a metronome, just sit down with a friend who has a watch with a sweep-second hand, and practice counting "ONE and TWO and . . ." as your friend times you. You should be counting a little faster than one beat per second, getting fifteen counts into about twelve seconds. Don't count beyond fifteen in your practice sessions; we'll see why in a few paragraphs.

To get a good idea of just how a 1½-to-2-inch compression looks and feels, first measure off 1¾ inches on a stick of some sort—a broom handle is fine. Find a fairly firm pillow or sofa cushion and press that marked stick down into the cushion so that the 1¾-inch mark is even with the top of the rest of the pillow.

Now lay the stick aside, form your hands as described above, and compress the pillow or cushion with the heel of your bottom hand so that it goes down the same 1¾ inches. It's helpful to have a friend handy to press the stick down right next to your hands, to confirm that you're really compressing the full distance but no farther.

Keep compressing the cushion until you can consistently press it down 1½-to-2-inches, stroke after stroke. Of course, human chests feel very different than sofa cushions or pillows, but the principle is the same; your own sense of how far 1½ to 2 inches is is most important.

(A word of encouragement: At this point, both the 80-compressions-per-minute rate and the 1½-to-2-inches compression depth are abstractions, even with metronome and sofa-cushion practice. But after just a few minutes' practice on a CPR mannikin, both will become very concrete and seem very natural. You'll be amazed at how quickly they become reflexive and automatic, like walking.)

In addition to compressing a victim's chest, we must also continue to provide a supply of fresh oxygen.

To do so, we pause after every fifteen compressions, lean over to the victim's head, reopen his airway, pinch his nose and reseal our lips over his, and give *two* more quick, full breaths.

To avoid getting tangled up in these numbers, let's go over them again: We give *15 compressions*, at a rate of *80 per minute*, then give *2 quick breaths* (which we'll call *ventilations*).

And then we immediately resume chest compressions, continuing the 15 compressions–2 ventilations cycle over and over until the victim revives or help arrives.

Figure 8-21

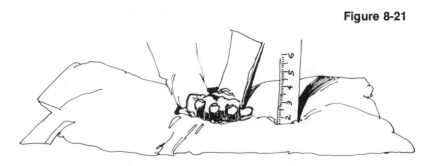

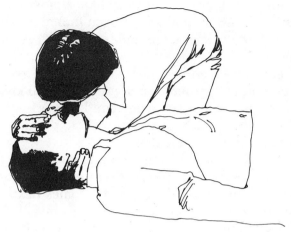

Figure 8-22

It's important to understand that for a victim whose heart has stopped, *both compressions and ventilations are required to sustain life.* If we only compress his chest the victim soon runs out of the oxygen that we are trying to get to his brain. And if we only breathe for him, the heart does not pump oxygen, via the blood, up to the brain.

For a pulseless victim, we always provide *both* ventilation and compression. Or, put another way,

artificial respiration + artificial circulation = CPR.

That's it: Now you know the ABCs of CPR!

And with that knowledge, you know how to save a life.

There are a few refinements you should know, and you probably have some questions about how and when to use these ABCs. We'll cover those in the next chapter.

For now, let's review the steps in the ABCs:

- AIRWAY—Open the victim's airway by tilting his head back.
- BREATHING—First look, listen, and feel for breath. If there is none, give him four big, full breaths.
- CIRCULATION—First, check for a carotid pulse. If there is none, begin chest compressions and continue breathing for him, at a ratio of 15 compressions to 2 ventilations.

57

For a little test, take out a piece of paper, close the book, and write down the ABCs. Explain what each includes. Give the rate and depth of chest compressions and the ratio of compressions to ventilations.

Don't continue reading until you're certain you know the ABCs. When you know them—and you *know* you know them—you also know that in an emergency you'll never fumble around, frightened and confused, wondering what to do next. The ABCs will guide you through each step.

Both in practice and in real emergencies, don't hesitate to talk to yourself, repeating the ABCs aloud, announcing what you've just done, what you found, what comes next. Talking to yourself in this way is analogous to an airline pilot's use of a landing checklist; no one's going to laugh at you. (Indeed, many of the most experienced rescuers, including those who must use CPR almost daily in ambulances and emergency rooms, talk their way through every time, to make sure they don't miss a step.)

One last point about the ABCs: Remember that you don't have to do the whole ABC routine for every rescue.

In other words, *pay attention to what you learn from the breathing and circulation tests.* If a victim is breathing, don't give him the initial four breaths; back up to the A step and simply maintain an open airway. Or if a victim does have a pulse, don't do chest compressions; back up to the B step and give him one big breath every five seconds until he starts to breathe again on his own or help arrives.

Some new rescuers become so enamored of the ABCs that they ignore what they learn from these tests, plowing straight through all the steps. Don't be a mindless captive of the ABCs; instead, use them as a tool to tell you what comes next and what's needed.

9 Questions and answers about CPR

Now that you've mastered the basics—the ABCs of CPR—let's add a few finishing touches and answer some of those questions you've been wondering about.

When do you stop CPR?

There are three circumstances under which a rescuer ceases to use CPR.

First, *when a victim's breathing and circulation resume spontaneously or he or she is fully revived.*

Second, *when help superior to your own arrives.* That might be a fire department rescue squad, an ambulance with emergency medical technicians, or a physician. (But don't lean back on your heels and stop CPR just because you see people in uniforms coming in the door. Paramedics have to unpack their gear, get out drugs and intravenous-solution bottles, warm up defibrillation equipment, perhaps establish a radio-telephone link to a supervising physician at a nearby hospital. If you're doing a good job, they'll want you to continue CPR until they're ready to take over. And you won't have to ask them when they're ready: They'll move you out of their way.)

And third, *when you collapse from exhaustion.* In this case, you're not really choosing to stop, of course: Your body is making that decision for you. If you cannot go another minute . . . well, then you cannot go on. But never make a conscious decision to stop simply because you think there's no longer any hope; you're not qualified to make that decision.

The simple rule: Go until the victim is revived, help arrives, or you drop from exhaustion.

What if the victim's heart beat resumes but not his breathing?
Good question.

After the first minute of the rescue, and every four or five minutes thereafter, make another pulse check. If you detect a spontaneous pulse, immediately cease chest compressions. Back up to the B step: Check for breathing. If the victim is not yet breathing on his own, maintain an open airway and give one breath every five seconds. If he is breathing by himself, just maintain the open airway until he is fully conscious and revived or until help arrives.

It's vitally important to *keep checking for the return of these signs of life.* We do not want to compress the chest of a victim whose heart has begun to beat on its own again; and we do not want to continue ventilating a victim who can breathe for himself.

Don't become so absorbed in the drama and tension of the rescue that you forget to keep checking for these signs of life in the victim.

What if a victim becomes fully revived?
What an exhilarating experience . . . for someone to literally come back to life under your hands!

And it happens. But as exciting and rewarding as the moment is, it can also be a very dangerous point in the rescue.

For very often, a victim revived by CPR announces that he or she is tired, feels weak, just wants to go home and get some rest. Perhaps he assures the rescuer that he'll "tell the doctor about this next time I see him." Or says, "I'm going to call my doctor first thing tomorrow morning and make an appointment to see about this."

That's dangerous—because that's where we may lose the victim.

You may have saved his life from that heart attack, but you did nothing about *why he had the attack.* If we know anything at all about heart attacks, it is that another may follow shortly, without warning.

How would you feel if you brought a heart attack victim back to life, allowed him to go home unexamined and untreated by a doctor—then learned that he had died of a second heart attack that night, in his sleep?

The simple rule: Every person whom we assist goes immediately to an emergency facility for further observation and treatment. There are no exceptions!

Do not lose, through failure to get follow-up care, that precious life you worked so hard to save.

What if I'm alone with the victim?

So far you've read two apparently contradictory statements: Always begin CPR immediately; but also, always seek help immediately.

If you are with someone who collapses with an apparent heart attack and there are others around who can be sent to call for an ambulance, the solution is obvious: Tell them to make that call, while you begin CPR for the victim.

But what if you are alone with a victim? You are in a huge, empty stockroom at work, say, and you come across a stock clerk, crumpled in an aisle? Or in a school building at 5:00 P.M. you find a custodian sprawled on the floor, unconscious?

Or, most frightening, you are at home alone with your spouse in the evening—and she suffers a heart attack?

You cannot waste time calling for help before beginning CPR. As you learned from the chart on page 20, every second counts in a rescue. *You must begin CPR immediately.*

If there is even the slightest hope of attracting someone's attention, cry out "Help! Help!" while you are shaking and shouting at the victim to make sure he really needs help and as you are opening his airway.

And when you think you're alone with a victim, count *very loud* on chest compressions. Who among us could pass a stockroom door, hear a bizarre chant of ". . . THREE and, FOUR and, FIVE and, SIX. . . ." and not peek in to see what was happening?

But if you are, finally, utterly alone, you must combine CPR with some scheme to get help.

If, say, you are at home in the evening, and your husband collapses with a heart attack, go to him immediately and begin the ABCs. If a couple of cries of "Help! Help!" are not soon heard and answered by a neighbor, think about the nearest telephone. Is it in the same room? In the hallway? In the bedroom?

Begin dragging him toward that telephone in small jerks, one each time you move up to his head for the two ventilations. Within a minute or two—or ten—you'll be close enough to the telephone to reach up, knock the receiver off onto the floor, and quickly dial 0, *while continuing the rescue.*

As you resume chest compressions, begin chanting "Help! Ambulance!" and your address: "Help! Ambulance! Twenty-one hundred Foster Road! Help! Ambulance! Twenty-one hundred Foster Road!"

Even if the telephone receiver is dangling or lying several feet from you, the operator will be able to make out your words and will quickly summon help.

All this must be accomplished without losing your rhythm and count on compressions, without interrupting and thus defeating the rescue. Once CPR is begun, it must not be interrupted for more than five seconds; you cannot call for help any other way without substantial risk of losing the victim you are working to save.

And if all this sounds difficult—dragging a limp body (perhaps larger than your own) twenty or thirty feet in tiny steps, keeping up the rhythm and count of chest compressions and ventilations, chanting your address without losing track of the rescue—well, *it is difficult.*

But it may well be your only hope of summoning help.

And the victim's only chance to live.

Another simple rule: Always begin CPR at once. Get someone else to call for help, but if that is impossible, find some way to summon help yourself, without interrupting the rescue for more than five seconds.

How long could I continue doing CPR?

That depends on your size and physical condition and your experience at CPR.

If you're small, weak, and out of shape, you might be exhausted and at the point of collapse in ten or fifteen minutes. A healthy young adult, in good shape and with recent CPR mannikin practice and good technique, might be able to continue for an hour or more.

But in a real emergency, these predictions don't mean much.

For when someone's life is at stake—when we know that we are all that stands between that person and almost certain death—we find a reservoir of strength and courage which allows us to continue beyond any reasonable, predictable limits.

No one knows how long he or she could continue a rescue unaided. Don't let the question worry you. When you need to use CPR to save someone's life, the chances are very good that you'll be able to continue as long as you're needed.

What about loosening a victim's clothing?

It's generally not necessary.

If because of a victim's high bulky collar you cannot get your fingers in position on her neck to check the carotid pulse, you should by all means loosen or remove that collar or garment.

Of if a man's heavy winter outergarments make you wary that you have not been able to locate your two-finger salute precisely atop his xiphoid process, then quickly remove those clothes.

But as a rule undressing a victim, or even loosening his or her clothing, is unnecessary in a CPR rescue. Every second lost in unsnapping or unbuttoning, unzipping or untying, reduces your chance of success at saving that person's life. You do not have time to fumble with a victim's clothing, unless that clothing really is impeding the rescue.

The rule: Never loosen or remove a victim's clothing for his or her sake but only for yours—because you cannot find a pulse or proper chest position.

What if there may be a neck injury?

If the circumstances of the incident—say, a fall from a second-story window—lead you to suspect a victim may have suffered serious neck injuries, you do not want to aggravate those injuries by lifting on the back of his neck as you press on his forehead.

Yet you must open the airway to begin saving his life.

In these (very few) cases, an alternative means of opening the airway, called the *jaw-thrust* method, is used. It is clumsy but no less effective than the neck-lift procedure.

To open a victim's airway with a jaw-thrust maneuver, simply place the tips of the first two or three fingers on each of your

Figure 9-1

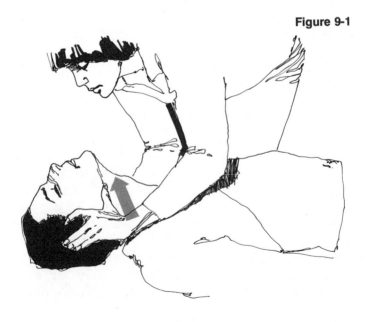

hands at the bony ends of the victim's lower jaw, and lift upwards while gently tilting his head backwards.

If the victim is not breathing and you must breathe for him, you will not be able to pinch his nose shut, since both hands must stay in place on the lower jaw to keep the airway open. Instead, as you seal your lips over his, lean your head slightly to the side and block the entrance to the nostrils with your cheek.

This takes a little practice; don't be surprised if you find it awkward the first few times.

And if you're worried that you can't quite get it, relax: Its use is rare; your chance of needing it small.

What if I can't get a good seal on a victim's mouth?

Although unlikely, it is possible that you may someday be called upon to perform CPR for a person—say, a victim of a terrible auto accident—whose mouth cannot be opened or whose lips may be so torn or otherwise damaged that you cannot cover them with your own.

In these rare cases, the rescuer attempts to seal the victim's mouth with the hand that had been supporting the neck—while

Figure 9-2

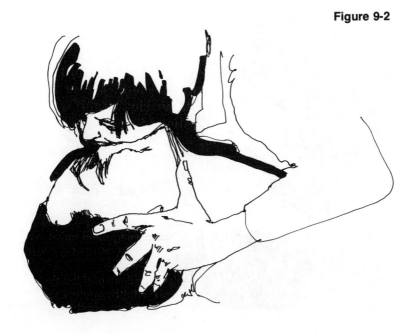

maintaining enough pressure on the forehead with the other hand to keep the airway open—and seals his mouth over the victim's nose for ventilations.

This is easy to learn, but if it sounds a little unpleasant, don't worry: Once again, your chances of using this method are small indeed.

What if a victim vomits?

Unfortunately, nausea often accompanies heart attacks.

And when a rescuer begins compressing a victim's chest, vomiting may well ensue.

If someone you are aiding vomits, quickly turn his head to one side, crook a couple of fingers and sweep the material from his mouth once or twice, return his head to the normal position, and *continue the rescue.*

Next time you ventilate the victim you may find you have to blow very hard, to clear the airway of remaining vomitus. Rescuers often worry that in so doing, they may damage the victim by

Figure 9-3

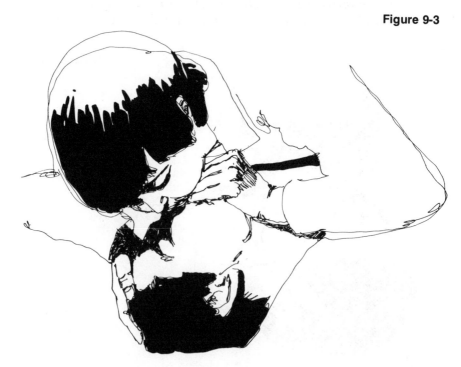

blowing the material into his or her lungs. The maneuver *will* move the material into the lungs, but the problem is not so serious.

Physicians know just what to do to remove foreign material from the lungs of a successfully resuscitated person; but they can do nothing for a dead person. Foreign matter in the lungs is the small price we sometimes have to pay for saving someone's life.

All this talk about the possibility of a victim vomiting during a rescue is very unsettling for most of us. It *is* an unpleasant, gruesome, unnerving experience for the rescuer. Even physicians, nurses and paramedics accustomed to dealing with messy situations sometimes find that a victim's vomiting leads to nausea in themselves. They occasionally vomit themselves when that happens.

If that happens to you—if you feel nausea sweeping over you when a victim vomits during a rescue—simply turn your head to one side, expel the vomitus, then force yourself to focus on the rescue and your life-or-death role.

You'll find the strength to continue.

What if I'm not sure whether there is a pulse?
Assuming you've practiced finding carotid pulses until you can almost do it in your sleep, trust yourself in a rescue.

All of us have had the experience of "creating" something that's not really there, because we wanted so much to find it, for it to be so. That sometimes happens in CPR: A rescuer wants so much to find a pulse in a victim, to avoid having to do chest compressions and also as a sign that the victim is really better off than he seems, that he imagines he feels a pulse when there is none.

The last simple rule: If you think there's no pulse or you're not sure, proceed with the chest compressions. Given well-trained rescuers, the greater danger for victims usually lies in NOT doing CPR.

How do I use CPR for smoke inhalation victims?
Just as you would for heart attack victims.

Of course, you'll want to first move the victim far enough away from the fire that neither of you is endangered by the flames.

How do I use CPR for electric shock victims?

Again, just as you would for heart attack victims.

However, before you go to the aid of someone who has received a severe electrical shock, make certain the power is turned off to the wire or wires causing the shock. If that is not immediately possible, it may be necessary to move the victim by lifting him or her with wooden (or other nonconductive) poles. Sometimes a wooden chair, cane, crutch, tree limb, or other safe tool can be used to lift a hot wire from a victim or to drag a victim away from a conductive object.

Remember that a victim's body itself serves as a conductor as long it is still carrying the electrical current. If the victim is still "hot," do not touch him with any conductive object nor with your own body. And be especially careful about stepping in a puddle, even a damp area, which reaches to the victim: That moisture can carry the shock to you in an instant.

Although speed is as important in an electrical shock rescue as any other, do not needlessly expose yourself to the danger of suffering a shock yourself. You can do nothing to help a victim if you are yourself knocked unconscious by a jolt of electricity.

How do I use CPR for drug reaction victims?

Just as for heart attack victims.

How about drowning victims?

Just as for heart attack victims.

Of course, you must get the victim out of the water to be able to do full CPR, but it is often possible to use some form of floating support—driftwood, deck chair, or surfboard—to support the victim while you (or another) paddle him toward the shore. When this is possible, open the airway and begin ventilations as soon as the victim is placed on the support, headed for the shore, bank, or side of the pool.

Very many drowning victims require only ventilations; often, especially if they have not been under the water for very long, their hearts are still beating.

Rescuers often find another anomaly in drowning victims. A person who has been in very cold water may still be resusciable long after the usual four-to-six minute interval after onset of unconsciousness, cessation of breathing, and circulation.

This is explained by the phenomena of *hypothermia,* or the chilling of the body in very cold water. The body seems to die much more slowly when it is thoroughly chilled. Physicians have reported cases of victims pulled from icy waters following immersion for as long as forty minutes becoming fully resuscitated, without memory loss or other impairment.

What if someone else there knows CPR? Can we do it together?
Thought you'd never ask. See the next chapter.

10 Two-person rescues

When two CPR-trained persons are present when a victim collapses, one can begin the rescue while the other calls for an ambulance. With help on the way, the second rescuer joins the rescue, taking over responsibility for ventilations.

If, however, a second CPR-trained person comes upon someone already performing CPR for a victim, he must first make certain help has been summoned, make that call if necessary, then return, indicate that help is coming, and join the rescue—again, by handling ventilations.

And when a second rescuer comes upon the scene, he must be careful not to interrupt or confuse the first rescuer as he asks if an ambulance has been called. A typical conversation might go like this:

Second Rescuer: "Has someone called for an ambulance?"

First Rescuer: "NINE and TEN and NO! and TWELVE and . . ."

71

Second Rescuer: "I'll go call." [He finds nearest telephone, calls for assistance, returns at once to the victim.]

Second Rescuer: "Help's on the way. I know CPR." [He kneels next to the victim's head and opens the airway.]

Note that the second rescuer asked a simple question, which could be answered by an even simpler grunt of *Yes!* or *No!* There was no chatter, no interruption. Upon his return he reassured the first rescuer that help was on the way—good news, no doubt, to that tense, worried, probably tired person—and without waiting for an invitation indicated he knew what he was doing, knelt next to the victim's head, and got ready to go to work.

As the second rescuer joins the rescue, he should confirm that the first rescuer has been performing CPR properly. He should also check for return of the victim's vital signs. Both tasks can be performed simply and without undue interruption in the rescue.

As the second rescuer kneels next to the victim's head, he first checks the victim's pulse *while the first rescuer continues chest compressions.* Checking a victim's pulse while someone is compressing his chest does not tell us whether the victim's heart has started beating on its own—compressions must be stopped to make that check—but it *does* confirm the new rescuer's visual impression that the first rescuer is compressing the chest properly.

If the second rescuer detects a pulse—indicating that the first rescuer is giving adequate chest compressions—he then calls out "Stop for a pulse check!"

With the first rescuer's hands *off the victim's chest,* any continuing sign of a pulse indicates that the victim's heart has begun to beat on its own and, of course, means chest compressions should not be resumed.

The new rescuer should also check for breathing. If the victim has not yet begun to breathe on his own, ventilations should be continued. If the victim *has* begun to breathe, neither compressions nor ventilations should be given, but both rescuers should stand by, constantly checking life signs, alert to the possibility that the rescue might need to be resumed.

If, after the first rescuer stops compressing the victim's chest, no spontaneous pulse is detected within five seconds, the second rescuer says "No pulse; do CPR!". He then immediately gives the victim one full breath, and the first rescuer repositions his hands on the victim's chest and resumes compressions. (The rate of compressions, and the ratio of compressions to ventilations, is different in one- and two-person rescues; when the compressor resumes chest compressions, he performs them at the two-person rate of sixty per minute. See below.)

What if the second rescuer's pulse check, while the first rescuer continues chest compressions, finds no pulse— indicating the first rescuer is not delivering effective CPR?

The answer is simple, if unpleasant: the second rescuer must get the first rescuer out of the way immediately and himself begin correct one-person CPR if the victim is to be saved.

In many cases this can be done with an indirect, reassuring remark, such as, "You look exhausted. Let me take over for a while." A tired rescuer may be hoping for just such an offer.

Other first-rescuers, however, may be unwilling to relinquish their job. Having invested time, effort, and emotion in the rescue, they may feel they have too large a stake in the victim's survival to step out of the picture. After all, they're convinced they're *saving* the victim.

In this case, the second rescuer—certain that the help offered by the first rescuer has been inadequate and that the victim's life is ebbing away—must be firm and decisive in moving the ineffective rescuer out of the way. There is no time to explain the whys and hows or to attempt to correct the first rescuer's technique; the second rescuer must simply say "Let me do it. Your compressions weren't working. *He's dying.*"

Two-person CPR is better for the victim, for there are no interruptions while the rescuer moves up to breathe, then back down to the chest. And it's far easier work for the rescuers, since each handles only half the job. The pace is also slower and less hectic.

When two persons perform CPR together, they always kneel on opposite sides of the victim. The "compressor" kneels opposite the victim's chest; the "ventilator," opposite the victim's mouth.

The rate and ratio of compressions and ventilations are different in two-person CPR. The compressor slows to a rate of sixty compressions per minute as the second person joins the rescue; the ventilator gives one breath after every five compressions.

Thus *the rate is 60 per minute* (not 80), and *the ratio is 5:1* (not 15:2). Before reading further, make sure you have those numbers clearly fixed in your mind. Close the book for a moment and write down the correct rates and ratios for compressions and ventilations in both one-person and two-person rescues.

The compressor's job is easy in two-person CPR: He need remember only to slow to the sixty-per-minute rate as the second rescuer joins him. To help maintain this slower pace, he changes from the "ONE and TWO and THREE and . . ." count to "one thousand and ONE, one thousand and TWO, one thousand and THREE, one thousand and FOUR, one thousand and FIVE, one thousand and ONE, one thousand. . . ."

It is important for the compressor to match his counting to his strokes so that the changing *digit*—the "one thousand and *one*, one thousand and *two* . . ." is sounded exactly at the *bottom* of his compressions. The ventilator will rely on this in breathing for the victim.

The ventilator's role is a little trickier and will require more practice; but once mastered, it's even less work than the compressor's job.

The ventilator must get the single breath he gives into the victim's lungs precisely between the compressor's counts of ". . . and FIVE" and ". . . and ONE," and the compressor cannot slow down nor pause at that point to help the ventilator deliver the breath during this narrow slice of time.

If the ventilator bobs up and down between breaths, looking around and not paying close attention, he will not be able to get the breath in between FIVE and ONE. Instead, he must stay bent over the victim's face, constantly holding the airway open, constantly attentive to the compressor's count.

As he hears ". . . and THREE," the ventilator breathes in deeply.

As he hears ". . . and FOUR," he pinches the victim's nose shut and seals his lips over the victim's.

And then just an instant after he hears "... and FIVE," he sharply exhales, filling the victim's lungs.

The victim's nose can be released after each ventilation, but the ventilator must maintain an open airway throughout the rescue.

There's an easy way to practice this breathing routine. It's no substitute for mannikin drill, but by practicing this way a few times before going to work on a mannikin, a rescuer will find the mannikin practice goes much more quickly and easily.

Have someone count "one thousand and ONE ... one thousand and FIVE" for you, just as if they were compressing a victim's chest. Hold the back of your hand up in front of your mouth: You'll seal your lips against it and exhale, just as if it were a victim's mouth.

As you hear "... and THREE," take in a deep breath.

As you hear "... and FOUR," seal your lips against the back of your hand.

Just an instant after you hear "... and FIVE," blow the air out against your hand.

This makes what is usually called in polite literature "a rude noise"; but it is an excellent means of practicing the second rescuer's breathing technique. You'll probably laugh the first time or two; by the tenth time you'll have it down pat. Repeat the cycle another ten or twenty times, until you're absolutely confident you're getting all that breath out *after* FIVE and *before* ONE.

Make sure your friend doesn't cheat a little, to help you, with

Figure 10-1

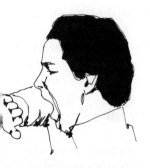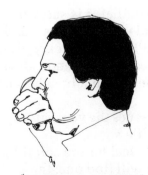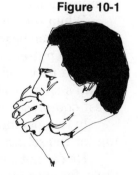

"ONE THOUSAND AND **THREE**"   "ONE THOUSAND AND **FOUR**"   "ONE THOUSAND AND **FIVE**"

a small pause between FIVE and ONE; tell him or her you don't want any extra time between the two counts.

It's possible for two rescuers to change positions without lengthy interruption of the rescue. This changeover is initiated by the compressor, usually because he or she has become weary and wants to change for a while to the easier, less taxing job of ventilator.

In the past, various changeover chants have been taught, along with elaborate procedures for allowing rescuers to switch positions without missing a beat. These maneuvers were hard to learn and harder still to remember and perform under the pressure of a real rescue. Recent research has indicated that as long as the changeover is completed within five seconds or so, such tricky maneuvers are unnecessary.

A much simpler changeover method is now used.

When he feels the need for a changeover, the rescuer compressing the victim's chest replaces his usual count of "ONE thousand, TWO thousand, THREE thousand . . ." with "CHANGE thousand, TWO thousand, THREE thousand, FOUR thousand, FIVE thousand."

As he completes that cycle of compressions, the compressor immediately moves to a position opposite the victim's head, opens the airway, and checks pulse and breathing for five seconds.

The former ventilator, having given the victim the breath due at the end of that cycle, moves immediately to a position opposite the victim's chest, and carefully positions his hands for chest compressions.

When the new ventilator is satisfied that neither pulse nor breathing can be found—taking five seconds for these checks—he says "No pulse, do CPR!" and quickly gives the victim a breath.

The new compressor, his hands already in position on the victim's chest, watches for that breath, then immediately begins chest compressions.

In two-person rescues the ventilator is responsible for checking for the return of life signs.

He cannot simply feel for the carotid pulse between ventilations, for of course he will find one: the artificial pulse created by the continuing chest compressions!

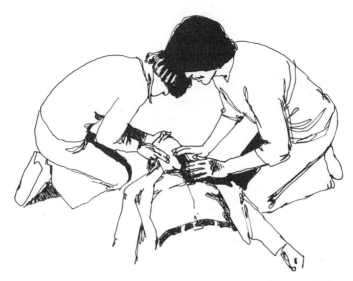

Figure 10-2

So instead, after the first minute or so of two-person CPR and every few minutes thereafter, the ventilator quickly calls "Pulse check!" as he finishes a ventilation.

The compressor stops for a few seconds—not moving his hands from their position on the victim's chest—while the ventilator checks the victim's neck for a pulse.

If there is no pulse he says, "No pulse," and the rescue resumes immediately. Time taken for this check should be no more than three or four seconds; it must not be more than five seconds.

If there is a pulse the team stops chest compressions and checks for breathing. If the victim has begun to breathe, they simply maintain an open airway; if he has not yet begun breathing on his own, they maintain the open airway and give one big breath every five seconds or so.

In either case the team keeps checking the victim's pulse every minute or so to make certain his heart has not stopped beating. Of course if it should again stop, chest compressions would be resumed at once.·

Another test for life signs exists and may be used in two-person rescues. But because it is ambiguous and can be misleading, it should be used only in addition to, never in place of, checking the carotid pulse and looking, listening, and feeling for breathing.

In this alternate test the ventilator quickly rolls back a victim's eyelid to see whether the pupil constricts as it is exposed to the light. If it does respond to the light, it is a good sign: The victim's central nervous system is coming back to life and the rescue is working. But if the pupil does not respond, it is not necessarily a bad sign: There are a number of drugs which might quite legitimately be in the victim's system that delay or reduce pupillary reaction.

Thus, this test is inconclusive and not a very useful measure of the return of a victim's life signs.

Reliance on carotid pulse checks and looking, listening, and feeling for breathing will give rescuers confidence that their diagnosis is correct, and that they will not overlook or mistake signs of a victim's return to life under their hands.

11 CPR for infants and small children

Because we usually think of CPR as aid for heart attack victims, and because we rarely think of children as candidates for coronary problems, few persons not trained in CPR would imagine the technique is used on children as well.

Wrong on both counts. CPR saves the lives of thousands of children every year. And kids *do* have heart attacks.

Generally, though, CPR for children follows drownings, electric shocks, smoke inhalation, and adverse drug reactions. As with adults, the same techniques are used for the rescue, no matter the cause of the emergency.

And CPR for kids is very much like CPR for adults. There are just a few simple differences and new numbers to learn.

CPR FOR INFANTS

Because infants are so small, we do not use the neck-lift method of opening the airway. There would be little room for an adult's hand under a typical infant's neck. Instead, it is necessary only to tip an infant's head back a little in order to provide a fully opened airway. However, if the head is tilted back *too* far, the airway closes down, for an infant's flexible windpipe can be pinched shut by excessive head tilt.

The best way to perform CPR on an infant is to hold the child along one forearm. One leg lies on either side of your upper arm, and the back of the infant's head is supported by your fingertips.

A simple adjustment with your fingertips can thus easily control, and if necessary, correct, the tilt of the child's head, assuring an open airway.

If you discover that your forearm is too short (or your baby too long) for this method, any firm, horizontal surface may be used for the rescue. A high counter or ironing board is especially convenient; performing CPR while leaning over into a crib is back-breaking and nearly impossible.

But if a countertop or other similar surface is used, a pad must be placed under the infant's shoulders, or effective chest compressions will be impossible as the baby's chest and trunk rock up and down, the neck acting as a hinge.

Although the arm-support position may at first seem awkward, the easier adjustment of the airway and absence of the need for a supporting pad make it preferable. In addition, with this

Figure 11-1

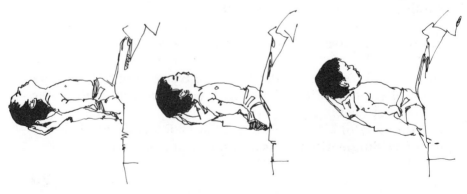

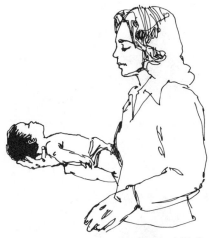

Figure 11-2

method the rescuer can hold the infant up close to his own face, making the rescue much less tiring.

One experienced CPR rescuer and teacher calls this the *football hold,* for it is very much like the way a halfback tucks the ball under his arm for a long run. Perhaps you'll find it easier to master if you remember that image as you practice.

With the infant positioned and the airway opened, we move on to the B step in the ABCs: breathing.

Check for breathing by looking, listening, and feeling for breath, just as you would for an adult.

If there is no spontaneous breathing, lean forward, seal your mouth over the baby's mouth *and nose,* and give four gentle *puffs* of air.

Figure 11-3

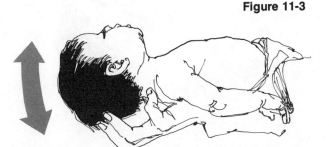

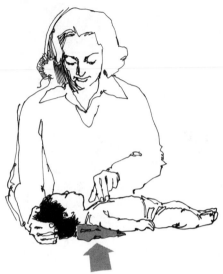

Figure 11-4

Two important points here: First, since infants' noses are so small and so close to their mouths, it's impractical to attempt to pinch the nose shut while ventilating a child. You must be able to cover both their mouth and nose with your mouth. This will be much easier with your face turned at a 90 degree angle to the

Figure 11-5

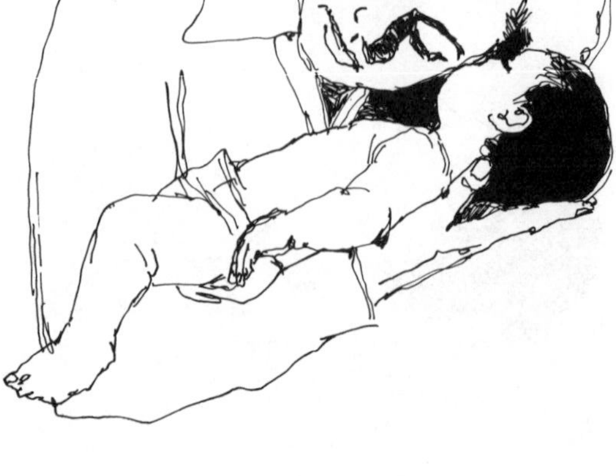

infant's, so the long axis of your mouth (side to side) is stretched across the up-and-down axis of the infant's nose and mouth.

And second, give only small *puffs* of air. A puff is defined as that amount of air already in your mouth (*not* your mouth and lungs!) without any special effort to inhale first. Infants' lungs are very small, and it's easy to overinflate a baby by blowing too hard.

With B complete, we move on to C: circulation.

We do not search for a carotid pulse in an infant's neck, but instead find it at his left nipple. The nipple lies over a portion of the heart, and with so little flesh and bony structure in an infant's chest, it's easy to find a pulse, if present, by placing two fingers atop the left nipple and pressing down very gently.

If there is a pulse, back up to the B step: Maintain the open airway and give the infant one more puff of air every *three* seconds.

If there is no pulse, chest compressions are needed.

Without lifting your fingers from the chest, slide them across from the nipple to the center of the chest. Imagine a line drawn

Figure 11-6

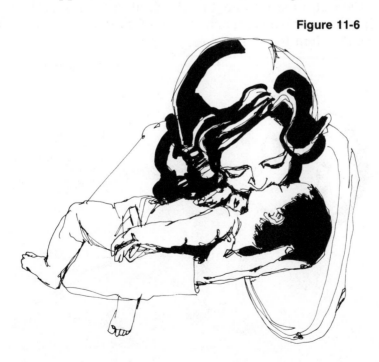

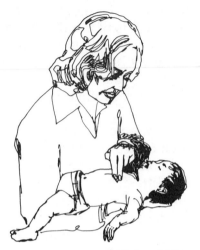

Figure 11-7

from nipple to nipple, and another drawn straight down the center of the infant's chest. Your fingers should be placed at the intersection of these two lines.

Using those two fingers, begin compressing the chest about 80 to 100 times per minute, to a depth of ½ to ¾ of an inch.

In other words, *chest compressions for infants are both faster and gentler than for adults.*

Figure 11-8

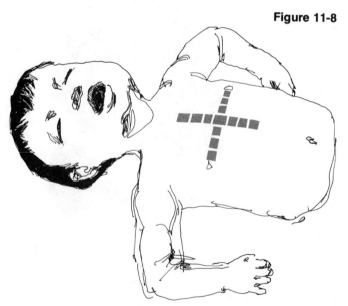

84

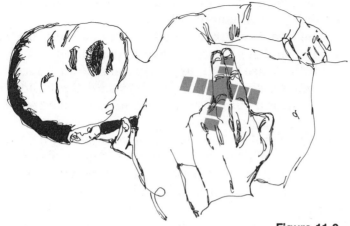

Figure 11-9

It's easy to get the faster rate down pat, using a metronome or counting aloud while a friend times you. Use a "ONE and TWO and THREE and . . ." count; you should be able to get about twenty ONE-through-FIVE cycles into one minute.

To get a sense of the correct compression depth, practice compressions on the inside of your forearm. Cock your wrist back slightly and compress with two fingers about three inches from your wrist.

The resistance of your forearm at that point is remarkably like that of an infant's chest. You can get excellent practice in both the depth and rhythm of chest compressions for an infant by using your own forearm.

Figure 11-10

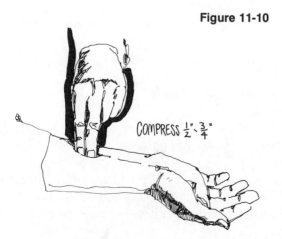

COMPRESS $\frac{1}{2}$" - $\frac{3}{4}$"

As with adults, we must continue ventilations on infants while providing chest compressions.

Give the infant one more quick puff of air, your lips sealed over his mouth and nose, between every five compressions. There should be little pause for these ventilations. Your fingers never leave the infant's chest; simply lean toward the child's head, cover his mouth and nose with your mouth, and give a quick puff. Resume compressions immediately.

Take only about as long as one of your standard counts for these ventilations. That is, your count should go "ONE and TWO and THREE and FOUR and FIVE and BREATHE and ONE and TWO and . . ."— except, of course, that *breathe* would be inaudible.

It's difficult to count at a rate of 80 to 100 beats per minute, while keeping track of the rescue, without mumbling. Mumbling is just fine, as long as *you* know what those almost undecipherable grunts mean. Most rescuers find their counts sound like this: "UNH an' OOH an' HREE an' HOR an' HI . . . UNH an' OOH an' HREE an'. . . ."

It looks funny on paper—in fact, it sounds funny when you do it—but who cares? *You're saving a child's life.*

Remember to stop every few minutes to check for the return of life signs, and to discontinue compressions, breathing, or both, if the infant resumes those processes on his own.

> Important: Skillful CPR for infants, as for adults, requires mannikin practice. Most organizations teaching CPR use special, infant-sized mannikins to give rescuers an accurate feel for the steps involved in saving a young life. *Mannikin practice is essential!*
>
> And *never, never practice CPR on an infant who does not need it!*

CPR FOR SMALL CHILDREN

If CPR for infants is much gentler than for adults, then CPR for small children is about halfway between infant and adult techniques.

You cannot hold a small child on your forearm, so a hard, horizontal support, such as a table or the floor, is used. However, as with infants a pad or other support is required under the shoulders.

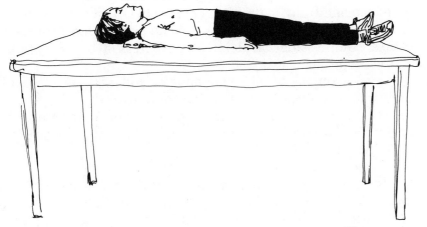

Figure 11-11

Open a small child's airway just as you would an adult's.

Check for breathing as for an adult, looking, listening, and feeling for exhaled air. If there is no breathing, pinch the nose shut, seal your lips over the child's, and give four *mouthfuls* of air.

A *mouthful* of air is somewhat larger than the *puff* used for infants, but much less than a complete emptying of your lungs. Try inhaling once, imagining that you are filling your mouth *only*, not your lungs. Exhale and try again. That's a mouthful.

Check the child's carotid pulse, and if a pulse is present, return to his head, maintain an open airway, and give another mouthful of air every five seconds.

Figure 11-12

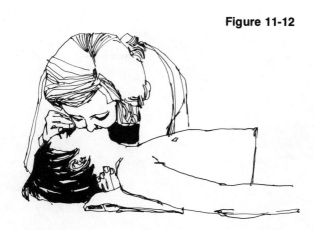

If there is no pulse, begin chest compressions by placing the heel of one hand *only* in the center of the chest, at the intersection of those same two imaginary lines used for positioning the fingers for chest compressions on an infant. Compress 80 times per minute, to a depth of ¾ to 1½ inches.

Once again, the count is "ONE and TWO and THREE and . . ." and a ventilation is given after each five compressions.

Remember to continue to check periodically for the return of life signs and to discontinue those parts of the rescue the child is able to resume for himself.

You may be wondering just how to differentiate between an "infant" and a "small child" for purposes of CPR or, for that matter, between a "small child" and a child large enough to receive CPR as for an adult.

Recently published standards have attempted to resolve the dilemma by defining—for the purposes of administering CPR—an infant as a child under one year of age and a small child as a child between one and eight years of age. Children older than eight are to be treated as adults.

Of course, any such rule of thumb must be tempered by the rescuer's judgement. A small thirteen-month-old child might well be treated as an infant, and a very small and slight nine-year-old might be treated as a small child.

Figure 11-13

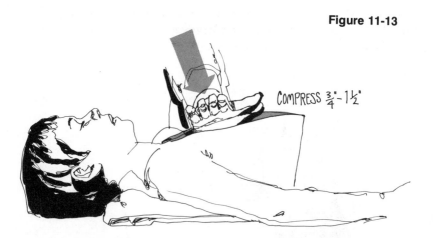

COMPRESS ¾"- 1½"

12 A quick review

That's it: There are no more numbers, rates, ratios, compression depths, or other facts to learn about performing CPR.

See, it really *was* simpler than you thought.

Before we continue let's go over a quick review of the facts you need to remember to perform CPR properly.

THE ABCS

In every rescue we use the little memory-jogging phrase, *the ABCs of CPR*, to lead us through the procedure.

A stands for airway; B for breathing; C for circulation. Here are the steps:

A *Open the airway.*

B *Check for breathing.*
If no breath, give four breaths.

C *Check for pulse.*
If no pulse, begin chest compressions and continue giving breaths.

Remember to keep checking for the return of life signs!

THE NUMBERS

Perhaps the easiest way to remember the numbers in CPR is with a little chart like the following. Study it for a few moments, relate the numbers to what you've read about each kind of rescue, then close the book and draw the chart from memory. When you finish this book, try drawing it again.

Here are the numbers you need to know:

		Victim	
	Adult	Small Child	Infant
Chest Compression Depth	1½-2″	¾-1½″	½-¾″
Chest Compression Rate	80/min.	80/min.	80-100min.
Compression-Ventilation Ratio	15:2	5:1	5:1
Amount of Air	lots	mouthful	puff

And, for two-person rescues, just two more numbers:

Chest Compression Rate	60/min.
Compression-Ventilation Ratio	5:1

13 Good Samaritan laws

Many new CPR rescuers ask what would happen to them if someone they aided did not live, and a bystander or relative of the victim thought the rescuer had done harm to the deceased.

And, some ask, what if they actually do make a mistake—say, compress the chest too hard, possibly breaking a rib?

What is your legal standing when you use CPR?

In an effort to protect those who give aid in emergencies, as well as to encourage such acts by qualified persons, every state in the United States now has adopted some form of what is generally known as "Good Samaritan" legislation. These laws offer immunity from prosecution or civil liability for the qualified rescuer who goes to the aid of another in an emergency.

When you attend a CPR class and earn a card certifying your skill at performing CPR, you will become eligible, in a sense, for the protection offered by these laws.

The laws vary from state to state, however, and it is not possible to make a blanket statement about their exact meaning and coverage. For example, some older, now-obsolete Good Samaritan statutes may offer protection only to medical professionals, not trained laymen; the laws themselves, often carrying the further confusion of varying interpretations by state courts over the years, are sometimes unclear.

Most Good Samaritan laws are based upon three assumed tests. Those whose actions meet all three tests usually become immune to suits based on those actions, *even if mistaken.*
The three common tests are as follows:

- The EMERGENCY test: The situation in which the rescuer stepped forward to offer aid must have involved a genuine emergency, usually defined as a life in danger.
- The GOOD FAITH test: The rescuer must have acted responsibly; that is, he must have had some reason to believe he knew how to do what he was doing.
- The FINANCIAL REWARD test: The rescuer must have had no expectation of, nor made any demand for, financial reward for his services.

Thus, rescues undertaken by qualified, CPR-trained persons almost always qualify under these laws.
You would not be giving aid if a life were not in danger. Your certification card from the American Heart Association or American National Red Cross attests to your skill in the rescue technique used. And you would not, of course, attempt to charge anyone for your help, given freely in the hope of saving a life.

If you want to know more about your state's Good Samaritan law, ask your family attorney for his advice. If you have no regular attorney, an inquiry to the local district attorney's office will usually supply the necessary information. Or write to your state's attorney general, asking for a copy of the statute and any relevant opinions available. If none of the above are possible or productive, write or call your state representative or assemblyman, who can at least supply a copy of the law and will probably be able to direct you to an authoritative source for its interpretation.
Local and state bar associations can also often help.

14 How to save your own life

Learning to perform CPR is a generous, selfless act: Since you cannot perform CPR on yourself, but only on another, your reward is your confidence that in an emergency you will know what to do to help.

You may well also someday know that satisfaction of having actually saved another's life.

But if, as you have read the preceding chapters, you have been wondering if someone will, someday, need to perform CPR on *you*—and if you find that prospect a little frightening, this chapter can help set your mind at ease, even help you save your own life.

CORONARY DISEASE RISK FACTORS

Just because the odds are better than even that you'll die from heart disease doesn't mean that you can't beat those odds. Attention to what causes heart disease and ways you can reduce, almost eliminate, your chances of dying from a heart attack can put you on the long side of those odds.

Medical research, especially since World War II, has focused at least as much on *prevention* of heart attacks as on their treatment. We now have a clear picture of those factors which lead, almost inevitably, to heart disease; and more importantly, we now know what to do to reduce those risk factors in our own lives.

Most researchers divide cardiovascular disease risk factors into three general categories:

- High blood pressure
  Smoking
  High-fat diets
- Obesity
  Lack of exercise
  Stress
- Age
  Gender
  Heredity

Let's call those three categories, respectively, *primary, secondary,* and *other risk factors,* and take a look at each.

PRIMARY RISK FACTORS

These are the Big Three heart disease killers. Any one alone can lead to a heart attack, but in combination they have a multiplier effect; so that someone with two major risk exposures may not have twice, but five or ten times, the danger of someone with none. With three factors the risk may be *twenty* or *thirty* times as great.

High Blood Pressure

All of us have blood pressure: It is the force exerted on our arteries by blood coursing throughout the body.

Blood pressure readings are written with two numbers, as 150/95 or $^{150}/_{95}$. The first (or upper) figure is the *systolic pressure,* the force exerted as the heart pumps. The second, *diastolic pressure,* is that force maintained between heart beats.

Physicians disagree on exactly that point at which blood pressure becomes too high, but there is general agreement that figures over 140/90 are cause for consultation with your doctor.

Oftentimes blood pressure can be reduced to a safer level by simple dietary modifications, such as using less salt. Failing that, or when the reduction needed is very large, medication is available which can control blood pressure, bringing it within safer limits.

If blood pressure is so easily controlled, it must no longer be an important factor in heart disease, right?

Wrong.

High blood pressure (or *hypertension*) continues to be a primary killer, thanks to lack of public understanding of its invidious effects, and also to that lazy streak we all share.

Few people know their blood pressure: How long has it been since yours was checked? Public hypertension screenings routinely find that a fourth or more of the persons checked have blood pressures high enough to send them to their doctors. So although we have the tools to treat high blood pressure effectively, we do not use them as widely as we could, simply because so many of us are undiagnosed hypertensives.

The lazy streak takes an even more tragic toll. Because the effects of hypertension are invisible—until that day when a hypertensive keels over with a heart attack, apparently "out of the blue"—even those persons who get accurate diagnosis and a prescription for drugs to control their high blood pressure soon stop taking the medicine.

They feel all right, they say: Why take medicine?

In one study in Baldwin County, Georgia, researchers found that a majority of those whose high blood pressure had led their doctors to prescribe medication had stopped taking the pills *within three months.*

Hypertension *kills.*

Undiagnosed and untreated, it is a primary cause of heart attacks. And hypertensives are *seven times* more likely to suffer strokes* than persons with normal blood pressures!

---

*There is widespread confusion in the public mind over just what a stroke is. We all see victims of strokes—persons who may have lost control over part of their bodies—but few of us know what strokes are.

When someone suffers a heart attack, his heart stops beating, and thus

How to save your own life:
Have your blood pressure checked regularly—at least yearly. Make certain your family doctor knows the current figure, and ask him what it means and whether preventive steps should be taken. If he prescribes medication, *stay on that medication!*

Smoking

You know all about smoking's role in causing cancer.

But you may not have heard so much about its importance in developing heart disease. A study at the Brookdale Hospital in Brooklyn, New York, showed that for every sudden death of a nonsmoker under fifty, there were *sixteen* sudden deaths of persons who smoked more than a pack of cigarettes a day.

Tobacco smoke in the lungs takes up space otherwise filled with oxygen and thus forces the body to work harder—the heart to pump faster—to get sufficient oxygen distributed to the body's tissues. And nicotine causes arteries to constrict, making the heart work still harder to force blood through those narrowed arteries.

Just as blood pressure can now be controlled, there is good news about the effects on the body of quitting smoking. People who stop smoking have only about half as many heart attacks as those who continue; and those who stop for five or ten years find that the damage is almost completely reversible: Their mortality rate falls to a level almost equal to that of those who have *never* smoked.

How to save your own life:
If you smoke, stop. If you don't smoke, don't start.

---

stops delivering a fresh supply of oxygen, via the blood, to the entire brain. If the victim does not receive aid promptly, brain death—the failure of the entire brain—ensues, and the victim is said to be biologically (or irretrievably) dead.

A stroke, however, is an interruption of the blood supply to one localized area of the brain. As with a heart attack, if the interruption lasts more than four to six minutes, tissue in that area of the brain begins to die. Thus if the area of the brain to which a fresh oxygen/blood supply is interrupted is that part of the brain which controls speech or the use of a leg or arm, that bodily function may be lost, although the victim may otherwise return to good health.

A heart attack leads to an interruption of oxygen/blood supply to the entire brain; a stroke leads to interruption of the supply of oxygen/blood to just one part of the brain.

Fatty Diet

Once, cardiologists' attention was focused largely on cholesterol, a fatty substance within the blood which seems to accumulate in the arteries, gradually choking them off in what lay persons call *hardening of the arteries* and physicians call *atherosclerosis.*

By either name the disease is a killer: When the buildup is sufficient, arteries simply shut down, leading to a heart attack or stroke.

Now, however, we are learning more about the other fats in the blood. More attention is being paid to new subdivisions of blood fats, high-density lipoproteins and low-density lipoproteins. It now seems at least possible that high levels of some kinds of blood fats actually provide protection against heart disease. We do not yet know what causes increases in these positive, protective lipids nor how to induce their production. That research continues and may someday provide us with a kind of natural immunity to heart attacks.

For now, though, the evidence is reasonably clear that diets rich in fats—from meat, eggs, dairy products, shellfish, and other cholesterol-rich sources—lead to premature heart disease and life-threatening atherosclerosis.

How to save your own life:
Ask your doctor about your diet. He can give you lists of recommended foods, other foods which should be consumed only in moderation, still other foods you should avoid—all in the interest of reducing your cholesterol intake. Get the lists, make up a diet plan, and stick to it.

Secondary Risk Factors

Although perhaps not individually so important as any of the Big Three, these secondary risk factors are by no means unimportant. They are particularly dangerous because of the ways they combine with one another and with the primary risk factors to produce lifestyles destined to lead to heart disease.

For example, fat people tend to get too little exercise, handle stress poorly, have high blood pressure and fatty diets, and often smoke. (What comes first in that sequence? Which is the chicken and which are the eggs? We do not know.) But when the obese shed extra weight they also tend to reduce their blood pressure, change their diets away from high-fat foods, get more exercise, and handle stress better. And now more conscious of their bad habits and the role of those bad habits in their overall health, many stop smoking.

Thus you can cut your odds of dying from a heart attack several ways: Determine that you will correct one or two bad habits, and you may find your reward is that you've made a dent in four, five, or more.

That is the hopeful side of heart disease mortality statistics: *Not only are the most important causes of heart disease easily within our control, but when we determine to make changes, each positive move brings on other beneficial changes.*

Obesity

It comes as no surprise to most of us that fat people have more heart attacks than thin people.

In one study in Massachusetts, fat people had half again as many heart attacks as those of normal weight. Other research indicates that the moderately overweight have a 142 percent higher mortality rate than those of normal weight; and those markedly obese have a *179 percent* higher mortality rate!

Obesity also helps lead to diabetes, itself another heart disease risk factor.

How to save your own life:
If you are overweight, get on a diet *and stick to it.* Avoid fad diets, which often actually increase dieters' weight through post-diet binges, and which can themselves actually increase heart attack risks (for example, through increasing blood cholesterol levels). Combine a sensible, moderate diet with regular exercise and you can't *avoid* losing weight.

Lack of Exercise

In his book *You Can Beat the Odds on Heart Attack,* cardiologist Irving Levitas has written that a regular exercise program is "second only to quitting smoking as a preventative measure to cut down the risk of heart attack."

That is so in large part because of all the beneficial side effects of exercise: Those who exercise regularly lose weight, handle stress better, bring their blood pressure down, frequently give up cigarettes and rich desserts.

Regular exercise also helps improve circulation throughout the body, increasing the heart's capacity and often leading to lower, safer pulse rates, while at work as well as resting.

But regular exercise doesn't mean a weekly round of golf nor pushing a vacuum cleaner from room to room. To provide protection against heart disease, exercise must be *regular, sustained, and vigorous.*

Most exercise physiologists and cardiologists say that at least three vigorous sessions of a half-hour to an hour per week are required for cardiovascular fitness. Running, swimming, bicycling, handball, racquetball, and other demanding, high-energy activities are often recommended. But if you're already out of shape and haven't exercised in years, a simple three-to-five-mile walk several times a week will work wonders; you can move on to more vigorous workouts later, as your condition improves and your doctor approves.

How to save your own life:
See your physician for a checkup, and discuss your exercise needs with him. Ask him to set up a schedule for you or to recommend a good local exercise program you can join. In many areas physicians are working with physiologists and others to set up cardiovascular fitness programs, which begin with complete physical exams and cardiac stress tests, then move into graduated exercise programs designed to build stamina and heart-and-lung capacity according to each participant's needs. But if there is no formal program in your area, you can do it on your own, following your doctor's suggestions.

Stress

Stress is a puzzler.

Many people who lead what seem to the rest of us to be exceptionally stressful lives show no evidence whatever of heart disease. Indeed, as we often say of them, "they thrive on it."

Because it is so hard to define stress, and harder still to quantify it, medicine is at a loss to assign its precise role in heart disease. Yet it seems clear that stress does play some role in forecasting our probability of suffering a heart attack.

Increasingly, physicians and other researchers are saying it is not so much a matter of *how much* stress we face in our lives but rather *how we handle* it.

For example, those who lead apparently stressful lives but are able to work off that stress through frequent, vigorous exercise seem to be much less susceptible to heart disease. Those who sit through eight hours of stressful work, then go home to plant themselves in front of the television set and worry over all those decisions they made that day, fall victim to the destructive effects of stress.

How to save your own life:
For now, we have no easy answer. The excellent books, *Type 'A' Behavior and Your Heart* and *Stress Without Distress* (see Bibliography) give details on ways of dealing with stress. A Harvard researcher has reported that meditation sessions reduce stress and probably reduce the incidence of heart attacks. Other studies point to vigorous exercise as the best means of handling that stress we all encounter in our daily lives. Today runners by the thousands—sometimes, it seems, by the *millions*—tell us of the joys and freedom of long-distance running, the falling away of stress and worries.

OTHER RISK FACTORS

These last three important factors are the ones you cannot do much about. Your physician will take them into account in developing your cardiovascular risk profile, and you should be aware of their implications, but direct action to counter their effects is impossible.

Age

Although heart disease is by no means any longer an affliction of the old—researchers report finding evidence of clogged arteries in adolescents these days—it is true that more old people die of heart attacks than young people. The older you get, the greater your statistical probability of suffering a heart attack.

But the only way to avoid getting older is to die: not much of a bargain.

Gender

Men have more heart attacks than women, so gender, or sex, is clearly a factor. But women's apparent natural immunity to heart disease has been reduced sharply in recent years: Since 1950 the ratio of heart attacks among men versus women has dropped from 10:1 to 4:1.

Some researchers attribute that change to increased smoking among women; others, to the emergence of women from sheltered roles in society. Both factors probably play a part.

And in any case, women's immunity declines after menopause, nearly catching up with men by age sixty.

Not much we can do here, either.

Heredity

For years cardiologists and heart surgeons have told audiences that the best way to avoid heart disease is to "pick your ancestors carefully."

If one or both of your parents suffered from heart disease, perhaps died from a heart attack, your chances of encountering heart disease yourself are substantially increased.

But in recent years we have come to see that the problem may be as much environmental and cultural as genetic. As Dr. William Kannel, director of the pioneering Framingham (Massachusetts) Heart Disease Study, says, "Families share more than genes."

How much of the role of heredity in heart disease results from poor dietary, exercise, and other habits ingrained in us when we are young? No one knows; it's a knotty problem, and we may not have definitive answers for another fifty years.

In the meantime, if you did a poor job of choosing your ancestors, you're stuck with them. And, probably, with some of their bad habits.

TAKING CHARGE OF YOUR LIFE

Though the figures on cardiovascular disease mortality seem at first depressing and hopeless, what we have learned in the last decade about prevention should give each of us new hope for our own lives.

Because we now know that the real answer to heart disease is not treatment but *prevention:* the adoption of sensible lifestyles, attuned to what we know about what causes heart attacks.

People who learn how to perform CPR often become interested in how they can avoid needing it themselves, and they find their increased sensitivity to the risk factors in their lives has a ripple effect: The people around them, the people they love and care about, work and play with, become sensitive, too, and begin changing their self-destructive habits.

Thus you have a chance not only to save your own life but also to take a hand in helping others—including those most important to you—save theirs.

For, as Dr. Kannel has written, "The fate of the potential coronary victim is, ultimately, in his own hands."

15 Telling others about CPR

Actually there are two aspects to telling others about CPR: telling your friends, neighbors, and co-workers that you know how to perform CPR and that they should summon you immediately in an emergency; and also telling those people and others about CPR itself, to encourage them to learn CPR themselves.

Most people who teach CPR agree that the single most important thing their newly graduated students can do is *tell others they know how to do CPR.*

If people don't know that you know how to save lives, you won't be called in an emergency. How would you feel if you learned that someone in an office next door to your own or on the floor below or in an apartment a few doors down died of a heart attack while waiting for an ambulance—because no one knew to call you to their aid?

You may want to write a simple note, explaining what CPR is and that you have become qualified to use it, run off twenty or fifty at a copy shop, then distribute it to the persons in your neighborhood, your co-workers, people at your church, civic club, elsewhere.

By adding the local emergency service telephone number to your note and encouraging people to post that note where they can find it fast in a real crisis, you may help save even more lives by helping someone call for help more quickly.

Make clear to your friends that you and CPR are no substitute for complex professional care and that you are not acting as a physician; but that your assistance may be able to save the life of a victim of a heart attack, electrical shock, stroke, smoke inhalation, drug reaction, drowning, or other medical emergency involving the heart and lungs through quick first aid until that more complex care is available.

See Figure 15-1 for an example of such a note.

You'll also probably want to encourage many of these same people to take CPR classes themselves. Perhaps you could speak to a church group, civic club luncheon, or professional or sports association, or other meetings, telling the audience about CPR and how you feel about knowing how to do it. You can help set up special CPR classes for the group. Your local Heart Association or Red Cross office will be glad to help and can even supply a speaker on CPR if you think you're not up to the job.

The ACT (or Advanced Coronary Therapy) Foundation has produced a splendid dramatic motion picture, "A Life in Your Hands," starring Burt Lancaster, which describes CPR training and encourages viewers to learn the skill. The film is powerfully affecting; audiences frequently have tears in their eyes by its end.

You can borrow this fifteen-minute 16mm color film for free to show to your group by writing to ACT's distributor, West Glen Films, 565 Fifth Avenue, New York City, New York 10017; specify your preferred showing date and one or two alternates. Your only cost will be return postage for the film after the showing.* Materials supplied with the film will help you publicize the showing and conduct a discussion about CPR afterwards.

---

*A special six-minute version of the film, suitable for television use, is also available; perhaps a local station would show this clip as a way of encouraging people to attend your session.

Figure 15-1

Friends--

You've probably heard the phrase "CPR." It stands for "cardiopulmonary resuscitation," or, simply put, the techniques for saving the life of someone who suffers a heart attack, drug reaction, electrical shock, smoke inhalation, drowning, or other problem involving the heart and lungs.

I'm sending you this note because I've recently taken CPR training, and I'm certified by the (Red Cross) to perform this emergency life-saving procedure.

And I thought you should know that, so that if you, or someone in your family, should suffer or witness one of these events, or come upon a victim of one in this area, you should know you can call me -- at 474-2131 -- at any hour, for help.

These emergencies require immediate assistance, so it's essential that you call at once.

And CPR is no substitute for professional care, so you should also call 357-9256 immediately for an ambulance.

Frankly, I hope you never need to call on me for this help. But if you do, I'm ready.

Sincerely,

Charlie Walker

Charlie Walker

MY NUMBER: 474-2131

AMBULANCE NUMBER: 357-9256

To make the most of the interest generated by your talk and/or the film, have someone from the Heart Association or Red Cross on hand at the meeting to sign people up for CPR classes in the near future.

The ACT Foundation also publishes an excellent quarterly newsletter, *CPR Citizen*, which covers new developments in CPR research, new techniques as approved by medical authorities, interesting CPR rescues, and other items of interest to those trained in CPR. Subscriptions are $3.00 per year (first-class mail) and are available from ACT, Basking Ridge, New Jersey 07920.

16 Attending a CPR class

Because we have throughout this book emphasized the importance of attending a formal CPR class and getting mannikin practice of the skills described in the book, let's take a quick look at what happens in a typical CPR class and how it can help you finally master those skills, confirming that you have become a qualified CPR rescuer.

As mentioned earlier, both self-paced and standard lecture-style classes are available in most areas, taught by persons trained by the American Heart Association and/or American National Red Cross and using materials supplied by one of those organizations.

LECTURE CLASSES

In these classes, generally covering four to six hours in one or two sessions, you'll see a short film describing CPR and showing how it's done. Following the film the instructor (or instructors) will repeat the demonstration and answer students' questions. Local emergency medical service will be discussed, and students will learn how to summon help quickly and accurately.

Students then gather in small groups around life-size mannikins for actual CPR practice. Instructors work with each student in turn to help perfect his or her CPR skills. There may be a separate area of the room with additional mannikins, where students can practice by themselves steps they need to improve before final performance-testing.

Elsewhere in the room another instructor may have an infant-size mannikin and will be conducting similar drill sessions, working with one student at a time on the baby mannikin to achieve satisfactory skills in infant rescues.

Students complete a short multiple-choice written test covering the facts and figures of CPR—compression rates and depths, compression-ventilation ratios, and so on—and also take a short, private *practical,* or *performance test,* in which they perform a complete rescue on a mannikin as an instructor watches.

Those who pass the written and performance tests—usually 95 percent or more of the class members—are awarded certification cards attesting to their skill. Students also learn how they can enroll in refresher courses in succeeding years to maintain their skills at a high level.

SELF-PACED CLASSES

Students in these classes often make their own schedules.

They may work through all the material, leading to their certification in a single day, or may choose to attend several brief morning or evening sessions or may schedule their CPR studies in other patterns fitted to their own daily routines.

At the beginning of the course, each student buys one or more self-teaching workbooks (a single, thick one from the Red Cross, at $1.95, or a series of seven smaller ones from the Heart Association, at about $1.75 for the set) and begins to work at his or her own speed.

Because there is no time pressure to keep up with other students, those taking self-paced classes may read and reread sections of the workbooks, test and retest themselves over material as it is covered, until they are themselves satisfied they have the information down pat.

The workbooks contain both factual information and "what would you do if?" questions. They frequently direct students to move to another area where they can view a film or slide-tape program.

At several points students are directed to check in with the instructor for confirmation of their progress.

When the factual material is mastered, students move on to mannikin practice—again, at their own speed. Instructors work with each student to solve problems and answer questions that invariably arise from the workbook material.

As each student feels he or she is ready, he presents himself to an instructor for the performance test, which is identical to that given at the conclusion of lecture classes: The student finds an apparently unconscious mannikin and begins a CPR rescue.

When all the steps, or modules, are completed satisfactorily, the student receives his or her certification card.

Those who have read this book will find themselves at home in either type of class—but way ahead of most students in their understanding and grasp of the material taught. Readers will probably be able to complete self-paced classes in much less than half the six to ten hours taken by most students. Lecture classes may take somewhat longer, since instructors may not be prepared to test and acknowledge the reader's skills apart from their usual class procedures.

Either way, you'll find great satisfaction in working with the mannikins, discovering for yourself and confirming for your instructor that you really have mastered the material.

And you'll be proud of that certification card . . . that little piece of paper that says you know how to *take a life in your hands.*

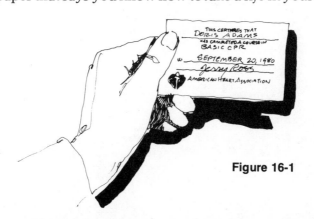

Figure 16-1

Bibliography

Want to know more about some of the topics covered in this book?

These books, pamphlets, and papers can answer your questions, provide background about cardiovascular disease and cardiopulmonary resuscitation, and help you understand better how your heart works and how you can help it work better and longer.

If the books listed are not available through your local library, check the current title or author volumes of *Books in Print*; these titles can be ordered through any bookstore. Publications of the American National Red Cross and American Heart Association are usually available from the local offices of those organizations; if not, you may write to the ANRC at 17th and D Streets, Washington, D.C. 20006, and the AHA at 7320 Greenville Avenue, Dallas, Texas 75231. The medical journals cited below will probably not be available in local public libraries, but copies may usually be obtained from nearby medical school libraries or by writing to your county or state medical society.

Cardiopulmonary Resuscitation. Washington, D.C.: American National Red Cross, 1974.

CLARK, DEAN T. "Complications Following Closed-Chest Cardiac Massage." *Journal of the American Medical Association* 181:4 (July 28, 1962) 127–128 [A study of common injuries caused by improperly performed CPR—mainly broken ribs—from the early days of the technique's use.]

COPLEY, DONALD P., *et al.* "Improved Outcome for Prehospital Cardiopulmonary Collapse with Resuscitation by Bystanders." *Circulation* 56:6 (December 1977), 901–905. [The landmark Birmingham study on the effectiveness of quick, effective, bystander-initiated CPR, quoted in Chapter 3.]

CPR in Basic Life Support. (pamphlet) Dallas, Texas: American Heart Association, 1978.

CPR/BLS Self-Instructional System. (workbook series) Dallas, Texas: American Heart Association, 1977, 1978.

CPR Saves Lives. Who Teaches It? We Do. (pamphlet) Washington, D.C.: American National Red Cross, 1978.

DE BAKEY, MICHAEL, and ANTONIO GOTTO. *The Living Heart.* New York: David McKay & Co., 1977. [A splendid examination of how the heart works.]

DIETHRICH, EDWARD, and JOHN J. FRIED. *Code ARREST: A Heart Stops/A Doctor Reports on the Battle Against the Heart Disease Epidemic.* New York: E.P. Dutton & Co., 1974.

Facts About Strokes. (pamphlet) Dallas, Texas: American Heart Association, undated.

FEINMAN, MAX L., and JOSLEEN WILSON. *Live Longer: Control Your Blood Pressure.* New York: Coward, McCann & Geohegan, 1977.

FLAX, PEGGY, *et al.* "The mechanics of widespread training of cardiopulmonary resuscitation. A community project implemented by volunteers." *American Heart Journal* 91:1 (January 1976), 123–125. [A report on a communitywide CPR-training program begun by American Heart Association volunteers in Marin County, California, in 1973, this gives a good picture of what happens in a typical CPR class for lay persons.]

FRIEDMAN, MEYER, and RAY ROSENMAN. *Type 'A' Behavior and Your Heart.* New York: Alfred Knopf, 1974. [The driven versus the relaxed life: how to deal with stress.]

GALTON, LAWRENCE. *The Silent Disease: Hypertension.* New York: Crown Publications, 1973. [An excellent discussion of hypertension: who, how, what to do about it. Probably the best book currently available on hypertension; eminently readable.]

GORKIN, JESS. "A Big Yes for CPR Courses in High School." *Parade,* March 5, 1978.

HASKELL, WILLIAM, and JERE MITCHELL. *"E" is for Exercise.* (pamphlet) Dallas, Texas: American Heart Association, 1977.

Heart Attack: How to Reduce Your Risk. (booklet) Dallas, Texas: American Heart Association, undated.

KANNEL, WILLIAM B. "Current Status of the Epidemiology of Brain Infarction Association with Occlusive Arterial Disease." *Stroke* 2 (July-August 1971), 295–318. [The standard work on the role of atherosclerosis, or hardening of the arteries, in causing brain infarcts, or strokes.]

———. "Preventive Cardiology: What should the clinician be doing about it?" *Postgraduate Medicine* 61:1 (January 1977), 74–85. [A simple discussion, directed to the family physician but readable by laymen, of what is currently known about cardiovascular disease risk factors and steps which may be taken to reduce those risks.]

———. "Prospects for Prevention of Atherosclerosis in the Young." *The Australian-New Zealand Journal of Medicine* 6 (1976), 410-419. [How to help your children avoid those lifestyles and habits which bring on heart disease.]

———. "Recent Findings of the Framingham Study." *Resident & Staff Physician* (January 1978), 56–71. [An excellent summary of the Framingham Study's information on what causes heart disease and how to avoid it.]

———. "Some Lessons in Cardiovascular Epidemiology from Framingham." *The American Journal of Cardiology* 37 (February 1976), 269–282. [A more difficult but more comprehensive examination of the data developed by the Framingham Study. Understandable by laymen.]

KOUWENHOVEN, WILLIAM B., and OTHELLO R. LANGWORTHY. "Cardiopulmonary Resuscitation: An Account of Forty-five Years of Research." *The Johns Hopkins Medical Journal* 132:3 (March 1973), 186–193. [A fascinating, readable account of the development of CPR by Kouwenhoven, the man generally credited as its principal developer.]

————. "Closed-Chest Cardiac Massage." *Journal of the American Medical Association* 173:10 (July 9, 1960), 94–97. [The landmark paper first describing the use of CPR to revive heart attack victims.]

Leader's Discussion Guide for "A Life in Your Hands." Basking Ridge, N.J.: ACT Foundation, 1977.

LEVITAS, IRVING M., and LIBBY MACHAL. *You Can Beat the Odds on Heart Attack.* New York: Bobbs-Merrill Co., 1975.

PACKARD, JOHN M. "To Thump or Not to Thump?" *Journal of the Medical Association of the State of Alabama* (November 1977), 10–11. [A straightforward discussion of the reasons for deleting the "precordial thump" step formerly taught to lay CPR rescuers.]

Red Cross First Aid Module: Respiratory and Circulatory Emergencies. (workbook) Washington, D.C.: American National Red Cross, 1978.

ROUSH, J. EDWARD. "911—A Hot Line for Emergencies." *Reader's Digest,* December 1968, 211–219.

SAFAR, PETER (ed.). *Advances in Cardiopulmonary Resuscitation.* New York: Springer-Verlag, 1977. [A collection of papers presented at the informal Wolf Creek Conference in October 1975 by many of the pioneers of CPR. The single most valuable reference work on the technical aspects of CPR.]

Saving Lives With Pre-Hospital Emergency Care. Basking Ridge, N.J.: ACT Foundation, 1977.

SCHECTER, DAVID CHARLES. "Role of the Humane Societies in the History of Resuscitation." *Surgery, Gynecology & Obstetrics* 129 (October 1969), 811–815.

SELYE, HANS. *Stress Without Distress.* New York: Lippincott Co., 1974. [A short, simple book offering valuable advice for handling stress in our everyday lives. Excellent.]

"Standards for Cardiopulmonary Resuscitation (CPR) and Emergency Cardiac Care (ECC)." *Journal of the American Medical Association* (supplement) 227:7 (February 18, 1974), 833–868. [The recognized national standards for performance and teaching of CPR.]

STARE, FREDERICK J. (ed.). *Obesity: Data & Directions for the 70s.* New York: Medcom, 1974.

What Everyone Should Know About Smoking and Heart Disease. (pamphlet) Dallas, Texas: American Heart Association, 1976.